JUST WHAT *the* DOCTOR ORDERED:

THE FIVE PILLARS OF OPTIMAL HEALTH

LAMIA KATBI, M.D.

DEDICATION

To every family I have ever guided,
you taught me more than you will ever know.

TABLE OF CONTENTS

ACKNOWLEDGMENTS

My story is not unique to me. My story is similar to so many professional immigrants who journeyed to the United States equipped with intelligence, hope, and determination. We all had one common goal: to achieve the American dream and create a better future for our children. I acknowledge your sacrifices and your successes.

Since I was a little girl, I dreamed of becoming a writer. That dream was shelved when I decided to become a physician. However, it never really went away; and as years passed, it kept poking at me from time to time. This dream became a reality with the help of so many great people.

In 2019 I came across the School of Greatness podcast, hosted by Lewis Howes. I started listening and I immediately got hooked. Lewis' messages about health and wellness resonated with my own. When Lewis and his team offered their first ever Greatness Coaching Program, I applied and was thrilled when I was accepted. I was the oldest person in the program, but that didn't matter to me.

The year-long coaching program helped me identify my life's new purpose: to finally become an author. I received the guidance and support I needed to hold myself accountable in pursuing this dream of mine. One person in particular stand out—Blaire Ward, the awesome team coordinator. An author herself, Blaire, helped introduce me to Alicia Dunams, founder of Bestseller in a Weekend. I started working with Alicia, and through her coaching and direction, I was able to write this book. I am so grateful for Alicia for pushing me and holding me accountable. I highly recommend her to anyone who wants to become an author.

Of course, I have to give a big shout-out to my editor Peg Moline, who was the perfect fit for this book and its message. Peg and I immediately connected. It was as if she lived inside my head and read my mind. With Peg's patience and encouragement, I was able to stay focused and committed.

Without saying, I am eternally grateful for my loving and supportive family. I am so blessed to be surrounded by so much love. My family is my village. The three people I want to thank and recognize the most are my children, Lana, Judie and Sami. Their belief in me, their support, and their love through this process has meant the world to me. Because of them, I want to become a better version of myself every day.

When the hospital I worked for declared me a 'disruptive physician,' I was devastated. Instead of firing me, though, they made sure I received the best care necessary to improve my health and supported my journey through burnout and recovery. I am especially grateful for the CFO at the time, Mr. Lou Molina, for his understanding and support.

I must give a special thank you to my team at work. As a physician, I spend lots of time at the office. My staff are my second family. They inspire me as much as I inspire them.

Lastly, I would like to thank my parents. My mom for always believing in me and my ability to achieve. My dad in heaven, who was an avid reader himself. My dad introduced me to the magical world of books. Because of him and his belief in me, this book came to life. I always wanted to make him proud. Dad, I wish you were here to read it.

PART 1

INTRODUCTION

"If you change the way you look at things, the things you look at change."

— Wayne Dyer,
author of *Change Your Thoughts, Change Your Life*

e are in the middle of one of the nastiest health crises in history. As I write this, more than 1 million Americans have died as a result of contracting the COVID virus,[1] which is tragic in itself. But what's even more tragic is that some of those deaths could have been prevented. This is not a vaccine diatribe, although experts estimate that 1 in 5 deaths could have been prevented with the vaccine.[2] This is a wake-up call: Chronic conditions such as hypertension and diabetes played a role in those deaths. The CDC reports that chronic diseases such as high blood pressure and Type 2 diabetes increase the risk of death from COVID by 18% and 15%.[3] I'll talk more about COVID later, but here's the thing:

To be healthy, one needs to strengthen the host. You need to strengthen your immunity, and change behaviors that weaken it, and most Americans are doing what appears to be the exact opposite. Check out these statistics:

---

[1] https://www.cdc.gov/nchs/covid19/

[2] http://www.healthsystemtracker.org/brief/covid19-and-other-leading-causes-of-death-in-the-us/

[3] https://www.cdc.gov/nchs/covid19/mortality-overview.html

More than 60% of American adults have been diagnosed with a preventable chronic disease such as heart disease, Type 2 diabetes, high blood pressure, sleep apnea, depression, anxiety, stress, osteoporosis, and infertility. These chronic conditions can be prevented, controlled, and cured through healthy lifestyle changes. Many are caused by alcohol and tobacco use, poor nutrition, and lack of physical activity.[4]

Heart disease is the leading cause of adult death in the United States. According to the CDC, more than 600,000 Americans die each year of cardiovascular disease – that's one in four deaths. Important risk factors include, again, high blood pressure, smoking, obesity, poor nutrition, high cholesterol, and alcohol use.[5]

Diabetes is on the rise: More than 100 million American adults suffer from diabetes or prediabetes, according to the <u>CDC</u>.[6] Diabetes is the seventh leading cause of death in the U.S., and the leading cause of kidney failure, non-traumatic, lower-limb amputations, and new cases of blindness. It's also a major cause of heart disease and stroke.

Obesity and overweight are big problems in this country. More than 40% – 250 million American adults — fall into this category and 360 000 Americans die every year from diseases directly related to obesity and unhealthy lifestyles. Right now, 17% of children in the US are obese, and in no states or territories are adult obesity rates less than 20%; three (Colorado, Hawaii, and Massachusetts) come close with less than 25%.[7] And because of these alarming rates of obesity, this generation of children may be the first to live shorter lives than their parents.[8]

Something's got to change. And I am here to help. I can help you because I have experienced failing health and have found the way back to vibrant, joyous health. First, let me tell you about my life as a doctor.

---

[4] https://www.cdc.gov/chronicdisease/about/index.htm
[5] cdc.gov/nchs/fastats/leading-causes-of-death.htm
[6] https://www.cdc.gov/media /releases/2017/p0718-diabetes-reort.html
[7] https://www.cdc.gov/obesity/data/prevalence-maps.html
[8] https://www.nejm.org/doi/full/10.1056/nejmsr043743

Chapter 1

SUDDENLY AWAKE

**"Sometimes you have to hit rock bottom before
you can start to heal."**

I'm standing in the center of a group of physicians. It's the culmination of nine weeks in a course for "disruptive physicians" and, yes, I'm one of them. There are a few of us, mostly men; we are led by a psychologist who moderates the session. In this specific session I was to present what I learned, how I changed and the steps I will be taking moving forward to prevent relapsing into my old habits, my old self — to prevent me from being a disruptive physician again.

The presentation included a written essay and storyboard. I had worked very hard on my presentation, and I was proud of the result. I wrote with dedication every night for at least a couple of weeks. I scrolled through hundreds of photos and I chose those I thought would represent who I am. I thought I did a great job, and I was excited to present. I wanted to show off my progress. I wanted to impress.

My essay was flowing, and I felt nervous but good. I had a lot to say and show. The words flowed freely and the more I read, the more I wanted to impress, especially the moderator who was leading the session. I was looking for approval and validation. My collage was busy, showing my patients, my friends, my family, and my life. The group listened quietly and started to give me feedback.

They were not impressed. Their feedback was objective, probably not what I wanted to hear. The psychologist who was leading the session was silent and in deep thought. He patiently waited until everyone finished commenting, then he looked at me and said, "You are the caretaker, you are the one who believes you need to take care of everyone's needs without paying attention to your own. You neglect yourself in order to please others. You may think you are taking care of yourself, but actually, you put other people's needs ahead of your own, ahead of your health and your life."

All I could think of standing in that room with my busy collage and my essay that talked about my progress and healing, was *Well, doesn't everybody put others' needs ahead of their own?*

The answer, obviously, is a big "No."

This was a big "aha" moment for me. I still remember how he looked at me and how quiet he was. "You are the mother of everyone." It was true because until then, I had no boundaries. And I didn't really realize all this until well after my presentation. I thought I had done well, but the only person who liked it was the new therapist, who complimented my writing.

But I had been brought to this moment, through this nine-week program, to realize that I was raised — indeed many women were — to think that my priorities were to take care of everyone around me. Everyone else. And what you find out is that it takes a toll on your health and your life. There's a price we pay. And there are ways to get through it. For me it took this program I was asked by my hospital to complete, this breakdown that, until the last three weeks, I wasn't sure was going to work. But it gave me the tools and I learned how to take care of myself.

You see, I now know my worth. It was a huge moment in my life going forward. This program at the Professional Renewal Center was designed for what was then called "disruptive physicians." Fortunately, that moniker has been changed to "burned out," but it's exactly where I was when I enrolled in a nine-week program designed to get me back to the great person and pediatrician I knew I was.

When we graduated from the program they gave us a token, a small bronze oval; we were given tips to stay focused, and they instructed us to use our breath. "Before you enter a room, take a breath, imagine a smiley face, breathe, relax. Anytime you have a moment of doubt or frustration, hold this token in your hand, and know that you are whole and that you are worthy."

The token was inscribed with three words: "Live with intention." I still have it, it is sitting on my desk at the office as a reminder of the person I once was, and of the person I have become.

I was awake. I was aware, which — when all is said and done — is exactly where you want to be if you want to pursue your healthiest and happiest life possible.

And that's the gift I want to share with you.

Where it starts

I have been practicing medicine for more than 25 years, and most of those years as a pediatrician, which means I work with kids and families — parents, grandparents, siblings — from all walks of life. I consider myself a mindful physician, an observant physician, and my aspiration is to help guide and hopefully change people's perspective on the meaning of health and fitness, diet, and exercise, and to expand their understanding of how to live mindfully.

There are many things that we already all know about. We learned them growing up from our parents, teachers, and coaches. We knew them by heart but might have forgotten, about exercise and how to eat healthfully. But there also are parts of the health equation that we need to be much more aware of.

I call them **The Five Pillars of Optimal Health:**

Sleep

Emotional Health

Mindful Eating

Intentional Breath

Physical Activity

And I believe we need to target them with awareness. I don't think anyone needs to hit rock bottom like I did to become aware and responsible for their health. But you do need to know, at a gut level, one thing: That you *can* take care of your own health, it is your responsibility — not mine or your partner's or even your doctor's — to take care of it and to learn about it – to always be curious about it.

Did you ever watch the TV show "Ted Lasso?" I was watching an episode with my son when Ted said, "Be curious." My son repeated it in the most meaningful way, telling me: "Mom, it's all about being curious." When you become curious you are willing to learn and later change.

Be curious about your health. Be aware and be responsible. In doing so you teach your children to do the same. Your children observe you and absorb from you, when they see how you take responsibility for your health by learning and taking charge, by seeing your doctor, by being curious, they will learn, too.

By telling you the details of my story, and how I turned around my health and my life, I am hoping to help you do the same.

Rebel without a job

I never thought I would become a doctor. Never crossed my mind.

I was born in a small Mediterranean city called Latakia, a port city in western Syria, born and raised. I was in school, getting good grades, but I didn't really know I was smart until second grade, when my teacher told me, "You know, you are a good student." I had gotten my first reward, a pink ribbon, and a book, and I felt happy and shy at the same time. I still remember my flushed cheeks and my surprise, and for some reason, I still remember that prize I got when I was six or seven.

I started reading and reading led me to discover the world through words. My dad, who is an avid reader, discovered that love in me and provided me with books non-stop, which I admired about him. My dad built an impressive library in our home, which gave me endless supplies of books of all genres. I became fascinated by books of most genres from ancient history to modern mystery books.

As I said, I never thought I would become a doctor. But in my country of origin, and in many societies, if you are good in school, you're destined to become a medical doctor, a dentist, or an engineer. Those are the top choices, otherwise, you are not considered successful.

But I wanted to be a rebel, basically, and be a writer. That wasn't an option for me because writing is not something that's popular back home, especially for women. There were so many taboos about being a writer.

The other option I thought I had was becoming a pharmacist, which required leaving my hometown and going to a different city such as the capital, Damascus. We didn't have a pharmacy school in my hometown and while I dreamed of being different, of being able to rebel and leave the comfort of home, I didn't have the courage to even ask my dad to apply, so I didn't.

At the same time, I knew my dad would be happy if I went to med school, as I would be the first in the family to go to medical school. In short, I wanted to make my family proud, I wanted to make my dad proud. My dad's best friend decided, "Lamia would be a good doctor." So, I became one. Seriously, I listened. I admired my dad and liked many things about him, but I did have a daddy issue — I always wanted to gain his approval.

So, my desire to become a writer never left my own head and was never discussed with my dad, as I was convinced he would not send me far away to school. Today I just wonder if those assumptions I made at such a young age were accurate.

I went to medical school and excelled there, I graduated at the top of my class. And I actually loved medical school. I loved anatomy, organic chemistry, and biology. I enjoyed attending lectures and learning about the body and how the human body works. I loved to learn. I studied hard and I loved literature, although I stopped reading and writing anything that wasn't related to medicine. I missed it and was hoping that someday I would be able to get back to it.

After graduating from medical school at the age of 23 with honors (medical school in Syria is 6 years; we do not attend college and we go directly to medical school after high school), I applied and was accepted to the top pediatric residency program in Damascus City. The reason I chose pediatrics was that it was the best residency program in the country, I knew the training was challenging and I liked to be challenged. I didn't realize until then how competitive I was. At that time I didn't realize that pediatrics was my actual calling.

That program was tough: On call every other night, and when you are on call you are up and at the hospital for 36 hours straight. It was brutal. In retrospect, I don't know how I did it for an entire year, and I still do not comprehend the logic behind the intensity of the program.

During that year a dream was born, a dream of becoming more, a dream of pursuing a residency program abroad. France was the top choice since many friends were there. But then another dream slowly made its way into the light. The dream of becoming board-certified in America.

Drawn to the USA

I met my now ex-husband in med school. He came into my life at a very low point, as I was suffering and mourning the loss of my first boyfriend of four years, a guy I met when I was 17. At the age of 17, I fell deeply in love with him and thought I would be spending the rest of my life with him, that he was my one and only. I was very romantic and believed in happily ever after.

When my boyfriend left the country to pursue his higher education in Spain, I fell into a deep depression. I felt devastated, but I was still trying to power through and do well in medical school.

My ex-husband and I started dating during the last two years of med school. He helped me get through the breakup, and I clung to him as if he was my savior. We had a lot in common. He was motivated with dreams to better himself, which aligned with my dreams. I felt life was giving me a chance at love and growth again.

We got engaged shortly after finishing med school. He had to serve two years of mandatory military service. As for me, I took a year off and worked in a village near my hometown, then moved to Damascus, and started my internship at the children's hospital. I spent that year being on call every other night, a year that taught me to be resilient and the power of pushing through, although I had yet to develop the tools and the awareness to know when and how to stop and take a breath.

Around that time, we started talking about where we wanted to go from there. We were shifting from going to France to going to the United States. You see, becoming board-certified in America was a dream for most medical students in Syria, but only a few can really pursue that dream due to many factors, most importantly, getting an entry visa to the United States. Financial ability was another factor.

We were able to speak with a few friends who had already gone to the US and who were either studying to take the grueling three-part qualifying tests required to enter a residency program or already had started a residency program, all of which gave us hope that we could do that as well.

Toward the end of my first year as an intern, we got married and moved into one of his family's homes. The decision was made for me to quit the draining residency program I was in and start studying for the qualifying exams. Our plan was once he finished the military service, then we would apply for our entry visas to the States. I truly believed it was going to work. We had fears about not getting granted the visas, but we pushed them aside and continued to work toward our goals.

We were advised — inaccurately as it turns out — to apply separately to boost our chances. So, we did, he was denied once, then his visa was granted. I was denied the first time, then the second time, and then a third time. I became extremely anxious and started to get depressed again. During that time, I became pregnant with our first child.

We made the difficult choice that he would travel. He traveled to Cleveland, Ohio, where one of our friends was living, and started to study. I moved back to my family's home in Latakia. I was feeling low and depressed, crying a lot, and feeling lonely despite being surrounded by a loving family. I remember feeling despair, worrying about what would happen if I didn't get the visa.

My first child was born while I was staying with my parents, and my husband was in Cleveland studying and preparing for his exams. The birth of my daughter made me even more determined to get the entry visa and join my husband, who had not yet seen his daughter. I remember how nervous, but hopeful, I was. I applied again for the visa, and it was granted. It was such a big win for me and our small family. I went from feeling despair to feeling hopeful and motivated to make a better future for the family.

We landed in Ohio when my daughter was two months old. I knew things would be challenging, moving to a different country, leaving family behind, and having only a few friends who also were busy studying.

Most importantly, I didn't speak a word of English. That's correct. I have never taken an English language class. My second language at school was French, and my French was limited. I couldn't attend English classes, as I had my newborn baby with me. I had to study in that tiny apartment we lived in, and I studied for the exam in English by translating the text from my native language, Arabic, to English.

I started to listen to the radio to get used to the language, I watched TV and found the courage to go out and just practice by talking to people. That first year was so challenging for me. I had to take care of our baby, study, and learn a new language, all in a brand-new country, in a brand-new environment, and, of course, with extremely limited financial resources. Those were difficult times, but I was so determined to make it, that I didn't pause to question any of it. I just kept going.

More than one kind of test

In order for a foreign doctor to practice medicine in the United States, they need to pass some very challenging exams. The most important is probably the ECFMG certification (Educational Commission for Foreign Medical Graduates), which is the standard for evaluating the qualifications of international medical graduates (IMGs) entering the US health care system, and it is one of the steps toward getting a license to practice medicine.

I studied for the tests in our tiny apartment in Cleveland, with my infant beside me. It was very challenging to care for an infant, study, and adjust to living in a new environment. But I did it and passed the qualifying exams. I became eligible to apply for residency but since I finished after the deadline to apply for the match program, I was only able to find a spot in an internal medicine program. I was lucky that someone dropped out and I was in. We needed to pay the bills and start somewhere.

I learned a lot in that year. I wasn't sure about internal medicine. I didn't know if it was a good fit for me. I found myself treating adults, many of them elderly, and that year was a very important one for me. I learned English during that year. I deepened my critical thinking and mastered assessment and planning skills which were very relevant in internal medicine since adult patients tend to have more issues than the pediatric patient population with whom I would soon be working.

During that time, my husband found a position in internal medicine in Chicago, so I started applying for positions in Chicago. I felt very blessed when I was accepted into the prestigious residency program at the University of Chicago in pediatrics. I moved to Chicago after finishing my year in internal medicine in Cleveland.

Dreams were starting to come true for us but at a cost. With both of us doing our residencies at the same time we had challenges finding childcare for our daughter. She was cared for by different babysitters (the cheapest we could get due to our limited finances). Then we put her into daycare where she often got sick, which meant one of us had to miss work, usually me. I started to get concerned about what to do. I really wanted my mom or my mother-in-law to travel all the way from Syria to help care for our child. When they didn't, I blamed them as if it was their duty to do so. It took me years to realize that pursuing my dreams didn't mean I could force anyone else to share the same view, and I couldn't expect them to leave their lives behind to come to help us.

So, we had to make some difficult decisions. I was in the middle of my second year of residency, in an intense rotation taking care of kids with cancer. Being the empath I was learning I was, I took it very hard when two children lost their battle with cancer. I felt devastated and overwhelmed, and I started to feel depressed and overwhelmed again. It did not help that it was wintertime in Chicago which I was still not used to. I didn't even know about seasonal affective disorder until someone in the program mentioned it to me and asked me if I was having "the winter blues."

We made the tough but necessary decision to send our two-year-old daughter to Syria to live for a year with her grandparents. That was purely awful, and I sometimes wonder if I ever really recovered from it. To send your child during their critical years of development, and not to be there for them, was one of the decisions I will always remember with a sting in my heart.

I still remember her beautiful face, her quiet smile, the way she held her purple Barney dinosaur so close to her chest in her blue OshKosh outfit, holding my friend's hand and waving goodbye without crying. It would be more than a year before we'd see her again.

She had a great time. She was well cared for, and she got so spoiled by everyone. To this day she believes it was a great year for her, and she never blamed me for it. I guess you don't need someone to blame you for your decisions, self-judgment is way too powerful.

And as hard as it was to let her go during such a crucial year in her development, in my heart I knew then — and I know now — it was the right decision. I also learned that many foreign physicians do that during their training; I know the idea was born after learning about another resident sending her child back home to India to be taken care of by the grandparents.

After more than a year, we were able to go and see her. I remember hearing her voice in person for the first time, speaking Arabic, and how happy I was. She was less than three when we sent her and by that time, we were well-adjusted in our residencies and were able to bring her home and find a good daycare for her. Life felt better.

Our second child, also a girl, was born at the beginning of the third and last year of my residency, and this time my mother was able to come and help us. She stayed with us for about nine months, which was great. It gave us such peace of mind. It was also good for the girls to have their grandmother with them.

During my last year of residency, I was asked to stay on for another year as chief resident at the University of Chicago, which was an honor. I struggled with the decision since we needed to start to look for work in an underserved area — inner city or rural — in order for us to become eligible for permanent residency and eventually American citizens. But I decided to accept the offer to stay, and I am so happy I did. I enjoyed that year. I learned a lot and I loved being responsible for the interns and residents. I was in a position of learning and teaching, which felt empowering to me.

With the help of a recruiter, the following year I was able to find a position in East Chicago, near Gary, Indiana, considered an underserved area, and only about 30 minutes away from where we lived in Chicago. I felt very lucky, as many of our friends had to move to rural areas to fulfill those requirements.

I worked at the local hospital there, the first pediatric clinic that was just starting. We started with no patients and within a few months, the practice grew exponentially. We brought on three other pediatricians in the first couple of years.

In medical school and during residency, I learned how to diagnose diseases and write prescriptions. During my first few years of practice, I learned how to communicate and how to look at the patient as a whole. I learned how to treat children and their families by observing the interactions between them, and how parents interact with each other. This is how I believe the mindful physician I became was born.

We decided to move from Illinois to Munster, Indiana, where we built our first home. We liked the area and the school system. Our last child, a son, was born there.

As I said, in order to become eligible for a green card, we had to serve in an underserved area for three to five years. I loved that practice and worked there for seven years, all of which were fulfilling. Then I decided to go into private practice with a friend from my residency who was also working for a different entity locally and wanted to go into private practice.

We joined forces and opened a beautiful pediatric practice. We became popular quickly, and very busy actually. The problem was we knew how to practice medicine, but we didn't know billing and management. We struggled in the first few years and then we started to have our personal differences. Our partnership didn't last, and she left, with many of the staff leaving with her. I struggled to keep the practice afloat. It was such a challenging time for me on both a professional and financial level. I was hardly able to keep up with payroll.

On a personal level, my relationship with my husband was starting to suffer. We started to have our differences and were seeing life differently. We started to drift apart. People used to look at us as the perfect couple – well-dressed, well-traveled, and very social. We hid our issues well. But eventually, we separated. Our divorce was finalized around the same time my business partner decided to leave. When I tell my story, I tell people that instead of getting just one divorce, I went through two divorces at the same time, which made things so much more difficult to navigate. The divorce was hard on us all. We struggled through it like families with divorce do. It affected all of us greatly. It took years of work to heal. We continue to heal even today.

It was during that time the migraine headaches, IBS, anxiety, depression, and fibromyalgia escalated to a new level. I wholeheartedly believe that the stresses I went through helped manifest those illnesses. I didn't know how to deal with life stresses, I was never taught how to, and my observation of my parents' relationship and other relationships around me didn't help. How can you seek improvement if you simply do not know how or where?

A new direction

There was an emerging trend in the U.S. Around 2010, hospitals started to hire physicians and other health care professionals on staff. The hospital would manage their practices and pay them a salary. Because of the costs of running and managing a practice, physicians were steering away from private practice. So, I approached the local hospital where I was already on staff. They assessed my practice and hired me and my staff.

I became an employed physician. I didn't have to worry about payroll. I had a manager and a boss. This was not easy for me in the beginning, as I was used to being my own boss, and I was into micromanagement (the mentality that no one can do it better than me). I didn't know how to delegate. I continued to want to practice and continued to want to be part of management.

It was difficult to let go of the little things. Conflicts and differences in opinion started to emerge. Some resentment started to build up inside of me and I didn't know how to address it. I thought management was not really listening to my concerns. Again, a challenging time. As I became more sensitive to criticism, my anxiety level spiked again, along with becoming critical toward the staff. Tension started to build up. I was the elephant in the room, and everyone was walking on eggshells.

The saga of illness

Through all of this, I worked hard, and I pushed harder. I failed, I got up and I kept going. I felt I had no other choice but to keep going, to keep pushing, to keep trying to prove my worth and what I was capable of. It was about me, about my own need to feel worthy and to feel appreciated.

When I was in my late 30s, I started to have dizzy spells. I didn't lose consciousness, but those dizzy spells became frequent and alarming. I went through many medical evaluations, from seeing a cardiologist to a gastroenterologist and then a neurologist. I remember when I saw the neurologist one of her questions was, "How often do you take over-the-counter medications?" My answer was "Every day I take either Motrin or Tylenol." She looked me straight in the eye and told me that my diagnosis was migraine headaches. I looked back at her and said, "Only migraine," and she immediately snapped at me, "Not 'only migraine!' Migraine can be a very debilitating disease."

And so, the long journey of treatment started. I had to learn more about migraine headaches and why I was affected by them. I looked at my family history and didn't find much, except that my mom also took lots of over-the-counter medications for head pain but was never diagnosed with migraine. Trials of medications were started. The neurologist also referred me to see a therapist who specialized in treating people who suffer from head injuries and migraines.

The headaches became more frequent, the anxiety that followed was intense, and depression followed that. At the same time, I was trying to navigate taking care of my children, my struggling young private practice, and a failing marriage. It took many years of treatment, seeing multiple neurologists at tertiary care centers, ER visits, and hospital admissions when outpatient treatment failed.

I started to suffer from a rare form of migraine: hemiplegic migraine, which resembles mini-strokes. I would lose the ability to move the right side of my body, and the ability to walk, talk or write. The migraines had this typical presentation of feeling nauseous and little dizziness followed by progressive weakness in the right side of my face, right arm, and right leg. That would last a few minutes or a few hours (the longest a few days), followed by an intense headache. Each episode would leave me very tired and feeling exhausted. And feeling helpless. During that time, I became anemic with low hemoglobin — due to gastritis and bleeding, most likely due to stress and frequent use of NASIDs — requiring blood transfusion, PPIs such as Nexium, and iron supplements.

Intense body pain followed, so many trigger points, so much fatigue, and so much trouble sleeping. And feeling defeated. More medications, more therapies, and more despair.

My illness also took a toll on my family. To see your loved one suffer and not know what to do is so defeating. I felt for my children at the same time, I simply didn't know what to do. It was very traumatic for my children. I know the emotional pain it caused them, even though I was and am still a great mother.

It was such a vicious cycle: The more headaches I had, the more depressed and more anxious I got. My body aches and fatigue were intense and vicious. My sleep was off, my eating habits were off, my activity level was off, and my breathing pattern was off. My entire life was changed.

I was on five different medications, so many ER visits and hospital admissions. One time I was admitted to an out-of-state hospital specific for headaches (the Michigan Head and Neck Institute). I spent three weeks there getting proper treatment. I had to spend Thanksgiving there. My three children came and visited, and we had our turkey dinner in the hospital dining room. During my stay there, my divorce was finalized, and my office partner decided to leave.

A closer look at migraine

According to the *Journal of the American Medical Association (JAMA)*, migraine affects an estimated more than 10% of people worldwide, occurs most often among people aged 20 to 50 years, and is about 3 times more common in women than in men. In a large US survey, 17.1% of women and 5.6% of men reported having migraine symptoms.[9]

People who suffer from migraine headaches are five times more likely to suffer from anxiety and depression. Furthermore, those with chronic migraines — defined as experiencing headaches on 15 or more days per month — are twice as likely to have depression and anxiety as those who experience less frequent episodes.

So, do depression and anxiety lead to migraines or vice versa? Most likely, it is bidirectional. I believe I am genetically programmed to have migraines and fibromyalgia, as many are (fibromyalgia affects about 2% of the U.S. population, approximately 4 million)[10]. I also believe that stress, inefficient and insufficient sleep, and an unhealthy diet were major contributors to the development of my illness.

It would take years of treatments to get my pain under control. As any desperate patient would do, I went to medical doctors, integrative doctors, and chiropractors. I was prescribed medications, injections, biofeedback, behavioral therapy, acupuncture, cupping, massage, reiki, yoga, and meditation. Many mentioned that I needed to change my lifestyle, but I dismissed that advice because I wanted to continue to push through. I'd had this thought embedded into my brain since childhood – that we do not quit, and we keep on pushing through.

Not until I was standing in the middle of that room at the Professional Renewal Center did I realize how important it was to truly work on changing mindfully the way I conducted my life.

---

[9] https://jamanetwork.com/journals/jama/fullarticle/2787727
[10] https://www.cdc.gov/arthritis/basics/fibromyalgia.htm

WHY I BECAME A PEDIATRICIAN

It's important to know why I'm addressing a general audience, but I practice as a pediatrician.

Children are our future, our base, our foundation. When someone asks you, "Who is the most important person in your life?" If you have children, you answer, "My children." To me, my children's well-being is the most important thing and I definitely generalize that to the people around me, my patients, and their parents. What we do for our children, what we sacrifice, is everything. We love them unconditionally. And if we want them to learn and grow in a way that they feel supported mentally, emotionally, and physically, if we want to create a better future for them, who is going to do that? The parents and grandparents. So, this is why, while I am a pediatrician, I also help families understand this and change the way they think and the way they deal with their kids.

There is a lot to learn by reading books and articles, and we have this wonderful tool called the Internet. But children also learn by seeing their doctors regularly, at least they do in my practice.

It's a family affair

I love the way parents are so committed to bringing in their kids when they are young to get checkups and vaccines. It's extremely important. Then, after the age of three, I only see them once a year. In the past, I noticed that it really dropped off after that. We just didn't see them. A parent would bring their children in only when they needed a shot for entering school, then maybe at age 11 or 16.

In our practice, we remind them and make the appointments for them before they leave the office. We say, "Okay, we'll see you next year," and also send reminders. These are **wellness checks**. I feel it's so important to be checking in with the kids, and with their parents, and teaching the children that this is something you do. And I make it a point to compliment my patients' parents who bring their children in for those checkups, not just for shots. I feel this will teach them how to take care of themselves in the future. And I listen to the advice I get from parents and grandparents and talk to the kids about that: that they have wisdom, they have knowledge, and they can give valuable advice.

There are now so many websites that one can actually learn from as well. I provide websites to my patients' parents in regard to starting solids, and which foods are healthiest for them at a young age. I would say the American Academy of Pediatrics (AAP), WebMD, and Harvard Health, all of those are great sources for parents. You'll be able to find resources in the appendix at the back of this book.

The path toward wellness

It all started during a day I was in such pain with a severe migraine headache, I shouldn't have been at work. I was working with a mother and dad who were first-time parents, and they required lots of attention. I could feel my headache worsening, the acid in my stomach rising, the dizziness, and the light and sound sensitivities intensifying. I was feeling frustrated and angry.

Instead of excusing myself, as I should have, I kept going and pushed through the more than one-hour-long visit. I know I was holding my breath. I know I was about to collapse, and I could barely move. After I finished with the appointment I made my way to my office and told the staff I needed to go to the hospital because I wasn't feeling well. I had started to feel the weakness creeping in on the right side of my body, the anger and frustration increasing in my chest and in my head. I yelled and threw my stethoscope to the floor. One person took it wrong and thought I was throwing my stethoscope at them. (Understandably so!)

I was then taken to the emergency room, but the damage was done. A complaint was filed against me with human resources, and I was contacted

by the administration. I was asked to get a full neuropsychic evaluation —
and I was asked to stop practicing until the results were in. I was initially
evaluated in a place in Illinois, and I remember not connecting at all with
the psychiatrist who conducted the evaluation. When I read the report, I
completely disagreed with their findings, especially since they asked me to
quit practicing immediately because they felt I was endangering my health
and the health of others.

When I was labeled as a "disruptive physician" I became angrier and more
resentful of the person who did the evaluation. In hindsight, I realize they
knew I needed help, and while I was totally in denial, I knew it, too. There
was no way for me to continue to function as I was.

I was never a big drinker, not until those stressful years in my life, during
which I indulged in drinking, mostly red wine. I didn't grow up in a drinking
environment and I didn't start drinking alcohol on a regular basis until I was
in my 30s, but mostly in my 40s. So that, along with a mild eating disorder,
was part of my diagnosis (more on that later).

Since I didn't like the evaluation (or the recommendation) I got from the
Illinois psychiatrist, I started researching where else I could go and found a
social worker who helps distressed physicians such as myself. She helped me
find the Professional Renewal Center program in Lawrence, Kansas. I agreed
to it, and I asked to start after Labor Day weekend since one of my children
was starting college. They agreed. The hospital paid for everything, and the
CFO told me he looked forward to me coming back — he thought highly of
me despite everything that happened.

I took an overnight train from Chicago to Lawrence. I remember being late
on my first day. I remember being sad, but I also remember being open to
learning. Subconsciously I wanted the help and I wanted to get better.

It was an outpatient program and we stayed in a hotel. It was an intense
daily schedule, with sessions from 8 a.m. to 5 p.m., five days a week. Hours
of therapy, private and group therapy, and a lot of assigned reading at night.

The participants were all physicians like me, from all different walks of life, from fellows to practicing physicians. The group at any given time consisted of six to ten people, with all kinds of issues.

I spent nine weeks there and it changed my life.

I already was into mindfulness, I was doing meditation (but not daily). I was already reading tons of self-help books. But we were assigned reading that would help us understand what we were going through; we read, then we talked about what we read in a group.

We read Brené Brown's *The Gifts of Imperfection*, and books about trauma like *The Body Keeps Score,* by Bessel van der Kolk. We read about relationships and about narcissism, and I learned a lot. *The Four Agreements* literally became my bible. Robert Sapolsky's *Why Zebras Don't Get Sick* explained to this high-power group how prolonged stress can cause or intensify a range of mental and physical conditions, including depression, heart disease, and more. Eckhart Tolle on mindfulness. All literally life-changing self-help books.

But what I also learned was that physicians are human. They do get burned out. And they need support, the kind of support we all need, and things can change with the proper awareness and help.

The program: Total breakdown

As many programs do, the Professional Renewal Center (PRC) program broke us down. You literally feel like they have slaughtered you and broken you down to pieces, broken down as a child might be. In the past, when I would see a therapist and mention to them things that happened in my childhood, things I still believe affect how I behave as an adult, I would be dismissed and most of the therapists I went to wanted to fix the NOW.

PRC was different. They asked questions about my childhood, my parents' relationship, my relationship with my parents, my siblings, my first boyfriend, and so forth. That was new to me, but at the same time, it was very intriguing. I always wanted to explore why we behave the way we do and what triggers our reactions. I learned that minor traumas cumulate with time, they become post-traumatic stress disorder (PTSD) and they start to add up.

So, we went through every single thing in my life. I remember listing them and there were about 16 minor traumas. One was the breakup from my first boyfriend, how he left me and the country, another the molestation I suffered as a young child, how I carried that guilt growing up, and how the family environment affected me, especially being a highly sensitive child, how I observed the maltreatment of an important person in my family, just to name a few of the things that happened during my early childhood.

That's when we were assigned to read Charles Whitfield's *Healing the Child Within*, which is all about why we do the things we do, and why and how we react to our childhood traumas.

Another book we were assigned was Viktor Frankl's *Man's Search for Meaning*, which uses the stories of concentration camp prisoners, including his own, for lessons in spiritual growth. To Frankl, it's all about keeping hope and a positive attitude no matter what is happening, we can't avoid suffering, but it's up to us to deal with it, find meaning in it, and move beyond it with renewed purpose.

There's a quote from Viktor Frankl that really spoke to me: "Between stimulus and response lies a space. In that space lie our freedom and power to choose a response. In our response lies our growth and our happiness." He lost everything, and everyone, and when I heard that quote it was such an eye-opener for me.

The Assassin

In our groups, we were constantly taught lessons that broke down our preconceptions. My first group session was run by one of the therapists everyone called "the assassin." He said to me, "Okay, you're the new kid. Tell us your story."

And I'm telling the group my story, how I was sent here because I'm a victim, that I was picked on and that I was innocent. I completely dismissed that I even was disruptive. And I was looking for sympathy from these people who I just met.

At one point, the assassin goes, "Who here thinks she (meaning me) is a firstborn?" and everyone raised their hands because most of them *are* firstborn. All of them are like me, super achievers, and hardworking perfectionists. They want to *do* something. But I said, "I'm not the firstborn." Now, I was the third child, but the first born for my mother and there was a seven-year gap between my older sister and me. So, I am actually considered a firstborn because of the distance between us. My next assignment was to learn about child placement and family ties, so I read Kevin Leman's book *The Birth Order Book: Why We Are the Way We Are.*

So, I'm in this emotional nine-week intensive that led to some powerful breakouts, and breakdowns. It was intense because while I was there, two of my foundations got challenged. As I have related to you, the two things I was most proud of and felt I had without question were 1) being a mother and how I was raising my children, my relationship with my children, and 2) my profession as a physician. It wasn't just about my reputation; it was my professional being as a physician and my commitment to my practice of pediatrics and my patients. So being called disruptive, a disruptive physician, was so hurtful to me, it was a slap in the face. I was being accused of something that gutted me. Both my professional existence and my motherhood were challenged. I was being kicked while I was down. And it was one of the lowest points in my entire life.

The therapists in the program were concerned about me during the first six weeks I was in the program. They had us fill out questionnaires every day and they were concerned about how depressed I was. I was never suicidal, but they were concerned about how down I was. So, the program that was supposed to last six weeks went on for nine weeks for me.

And that's when everything started to click. All the talking, reading, and meeting other people who were in the same boat as I was, something started to change. Something started to open up, something improved.

I started to FEEL better. I look back at the daily progress sheets we had to keep, and I realize I was not waking up with flashbacks every morning, my pain was lessening and yes, I was getting better.

Mood Survey

Name:_______________________   Date:_______________________

Please check mark to the left present symptoms you are concerned about. For each symptom that you are concerned about give a Subjective Unit of Distress (SUD's) rating to the right of the item (where 0=none and 100=severe).

PHYSICAL SYMPTOMS & EMOTIONAL CONTROL

_____ Number hours slept: _____ Rating: _____
_____ Nightmares _____
_____ Normal appetite *(circle one)* normal/too much/too little
_____ Feeling sad _____
_____ Tearfulness _____
_____ Feeling hopeless _____
_____ Feelings of discouragement _____
_____ Not able to experience pleasure _____
_____ Feeling irritable/anger/outburst _____
_____ Shame/guilt _____
_____ Short-term memory_____
_____ No concentration _____
_____ Not able to make decisions _____
_____ I feel overwhelmed _____
_____ I feel burned-out _____
_____ Feeling anxious _____
_____ Worrying _____
_____ Panic _____
_____ Tightness or tense muscles _____
_____ Shakiness _____
_____ Dizziness or lightheadedness _____
_____ Escalating emotional situations _____
_____ Hallucinations _____
_____ Shut down/numbness _____
_____ Feelings of detachment or feelings of unreality _____
_____ Stuffing _____
_____ Feeling sluggish _____
_____ Feeling restless _____
_____ Headaches _____
_____ GI distress (nausea, diarrhea, vomiting) _____

URGES
_____ Thoughts of death _____
_____ Suicidal thoughts _____
_____ Suicidal urges _____
_____ I can contract for safety for suicidal urges
Has completed a safety wellness plan? YES or NO
Safety Plan for today_____________________

_____ Homicidal thoughts _____
_____ I can contract for safety for homicidal urges
Has completed a safety wellness plan? YES or NO
Safety Plan for today_____________________

_____ Thoughts/urges to self-harm _____
_____ Urges to engage in reckless behavior _____
(Drinking, fighting, gambling, over spending, speeding, affairs, etc.)

ACTIVITIES & PERSONAL RELATIONSHIPS

_____ I have trouble being assertive to others. _____
_____ I have difficulty socializing with others. _____
_____ I have trouble feeling close towards others. _____
_____ I feel more callous towards other. _____
_____ I have trouble completing my daily routine. _____
_____ I have trouble choosing to leave things undone w/o guilt. _____
_____ I have difficulty planning. _____
_____ I feel anxious outside of my safety zone. _____
_____ I avoid uncomfortable situations. _____
_____ I have difficulty engaging in helpful activities. _____
_____ I have difficulty with procrastination. _____

Please mark if true in the last week:

__ I have not been able to sleep for more than two days.

__ I had decreased appetite for more than two days.

__ I had an increase in Panic attacks

__ I have increased tearfulness

__ I had an increase in hallucinations/flashbacks.

__ My nightmares have been worse for more than two days

__ I have not taken one or more of my medications for more than 24 hours.

__ I have started a new medication either Rx or over-the-counter

__ I have stopped my medication or changed how I take it on my own

__ I think I am having medical side effects. If so, they are: _______
____
____

Mood Survey

Name:____________________ Date:____________________

TREATMENT PRACTICE ACCOUNTABILITY

What relaxation (Mindfulness) technique did I use/practice last night:

____
(Deep Breathing, Deep Muscle Relaxation, Focus on Warm and Heavy, Guided Imagery/Safe Place, Holding a Stone, Ally technique, Music)

What Pause Technique did I use/practice last night:_______________

(Ice, Taste, Smell/Scents, 5-4-3-2-1, Music, Touch, Backwards Alphabet, Sing a song, Write upside down, Relaxation (focused breathing), hold the stone, One Minute Counting, Read Positive Affirmations, Read Meditation/Devotional Book, Review Positive Data Log, Tactical Breathing, Yoga/belly breathing,..)

What Treatment Responsibility(s) did I complete last night:_______________

____

____

How did I practice Assertiveness:_______________

____

How did I spend time with Positive People or Family:_______________

____

REFLECTIONS

What are three things that went well and how does it mean I'm changing?
Optional: Positive focus/Skill:_______________

    1. _______________________________
____
    2. _______________________________
____
    3. _______________________________
____

What did I receive today?
    1. _______________________________
____
    2. _______________________________
____
    3. _______________________________
____

What did I give today?
    1. _______________________________
____
    2. _______________________________
____
    3. _______________________________
____

What troubles did I cause others today?
    1. _______________________________
____
    2. _______________________________
____
    3. _______________________________
____

I don't think I realized until much later how important those few weeks were for me. They just changed my life for the better. And what was once the worst thing that ever happened to me became the best thing that ever happened to me.

It's what I want my readers and my patients to know, that they may be on the brink of a major health breakdown, heart disease, diabetes, and cancer. But stepping back and observing their health, paying attention, and learning from what is happening can get them through, and teach them how to have a healthy, happy life.

I can say truthfully that that program got me where I am today. Am I perfect? Of course not. But I am exactly where I need to be right now. I enjoy being in the now, as Eckhart Tolle wrote about in *The Power of Now*. It is what living mindfully is all about.

And I love where I am in life.

Back to life

I came out of the program, came back to the hospital, and started working hard again. There were some adjustments. At first, my salary was cut by 30%, and it took a few years to get it back up again and for me to get established in my area again. But I did and again became a popular practicing pediatrician, with many faithful followers. What was interesting is that I realized I didn't have to be there every day for people to love me and seek my advice. They respected the boundaries I set for myself to protect my health.

When I came back, I was trying to re-establish myself with the hospital in a mindful way, and I still had headaches occasionally. But I also had an action plan to follow. I had to see a therapist, which was very important — you didn't just leave and go back to your old life. I changed therapists a couple of times but found one with whom I really connected. I found resources to keep me accountable for my own health and wellness.

And I had an action plan for when I felt a migraine coming on. (See Lamia's Pain Management Plan, below.) Over time, I realized I wasn't experiencing as much pain, I was moving better, I was sleeping better, and I wasn't getting headaches as often. The burning sensations from fibromyalgia are almost gone now, and I can't remember the last time I had a hemiplegic migraine.

In retrospect, I feel incredibly lucky to have been in the PRC program. Yes, I was sent there, but I feel like I was given a second chance. And in this book, in the next chapter, I'm going to show you what I learned about awareness and how self-awareness can change your life, too.

"With everything that has happened to you, you can either feel sorry for yourself or treat what has happened as a gift. Everything is either an opportunity to grow or an obstacle to keep you from growing. You get to choose."

—Wayne Dyer

LAMIA'S PAIN MANAGEMENT PLAN

Prevention

    Avoid HALT (Hungry, Angry, Lonely, Tired)

    Drink plenty of water

    Sleep hygiene

    No alcohol, smoking, or drugs

    Caffeine 2-3 x daily, not at night

    Continue gluten-free diet

    Practice daily meditation and mindfulness exercises

    Yoga/weight training 3-4 x weekly

    No calls

    Regular massage

    Headache diary

Limit TV watching

Identify triggers

Take medication daily

Identify who needs to be notified of this plan, and where it should be posted, and send a hard copy.

Your warning signs: aura, fatigue, stress.

Your medication/access and administration: Toradol IM or Excedrin two tabs. Always in the drawer next to my desk and accessible to the nurses.

Water to be always present at this location.

Coffee at the start of any headache. Limit drinking caffeinated beverages in the afternoon/evening.

Approach: Find a safe place to go – my room. Lie down for 15 to 30 minutes while listening to relaxing music. Can try a body scan relaxation if I am able, and breathing/meditation techniques.

Reintegration: Start to see patients again. However, only I can decide if the episode is bad enough for the day to be canceled and patients rescheduled or sent to urgent care. Depends on their presenting complaint. Clinical staff will be able to make that decision.

Questions: Who needs to be notified of this plan?

Is it okay to administer Toradol, rest for a short time, then work again?

Is it okay for clinical staff to administer Toradol or is that crossing a boundary? Yes

Chapter 2

THE BURNOUT EPIDEMIC

"Burnout is nature's way of telling you, you've been going through the motions – your soul has departed – you're a zombie, a member of the walking dead, a sleepwalker. False optimism is like administrating stimulants to an exhausted nervous system."

— Sam Keen,
Fire in the Belly: On Being a Man

You probably have picked up on this from my story but getting that designation as a "disruptive physician" was one of the most hurtful and humiliating occurrences of my career, of my life. The two accomplishments in my life of which I was most proud were my success and popularity as a pediatric physician and being a solid and loving mother to my three children.

As I told you earlier, thankfully around 2018 the label changed to "burned-out" physician and while I fit some of the criteria of the "disruptive physician" — throwing things, excessive alcohol use — I since have realized that "burned out" is a more appropriate term.

I also realized I was not alone. The incidence of physician burnout is really prevalent. It's being recognized more than ever these days, and a big part of that has to do with the COVID pandemic. People saw how deeply healthcare workers were affected — emotionally and physically — by the endless hours and heartbreaking work they had to endure. I also saw many of my colleagues opening up and talking about the burnout they were experiencing.

It takes courage to open up like that, to admit to the public that we doctors are human. Because when you have to be in charge, when you are in a position of leadership, of authority, you have to show strength. People are looking up to you and need to trust you. You also are expected to show patience and poise.

In reality, the demands of being a physician can lead to high levels of stress. Even before COVID, a study by the American Medical Association (AMA) found that 45.8% of doctors surveyed had experienced burnout, defined as a "psychological syndrome characterized by emotional exhaustion, depersonalization, and a sense of reduced accomplishment in day-to-day work."[11]

A report in the *Archives of Internal Medicine* adds that "a loss of enthusiasm for work, feelings of cynicism, and a low sense of personal accomplishment" [12] also indicate signs of burnout. The interesting thing is that of all physicians reviewed, pediatricians were among the least likely to experience burnout (ER doctors are the highest). [13]

Since COVID, physician burnout is hovering around 61%,[14] and at the last count, led more than 3,000 doctors to leave their jobs. We feel it in my office, I feel the effects of COVID stress among my staff and among my colleagues and co-workers. We are short-staffed and so many people are on edge.

---

[11] https://www.ama-assn.org/topics/physician-burnout

[12] Maslach, C.; Jackson, S.E.; Leiter, M.P. Maslach Burnout Inventory Manual, 3rd ed.; Consulting Psychologists

[13] https://www.medscape.com/features/slideshow/lifestyle/2013/public

[14] https://www.ama-assn.org/practice-management/physician-health/half-health-workers-report -burnout-amid-covid-19

Another huge contributing factor, I believe, is the amount of bureaucracy and paperwork we are asked to deal with, again, often with a very small staff.

What doctors wish patients knew

Fortunately, so much has come to light about this, and I see the public responding very kindly and patiently. Recently, the AMA has been publishing reports about what leads to doctor burnout — task overload, patient dissatisfaction, feeling a loss of control, and diminished feelings of accomplishment — and it's a good thing because stress management and burnout prevention are not typically covered in medical school. What I went through and survived, and the treatment I got, turned out to be very grounding, and I'd like to help doctors to be able to cope with it.

I'd also like patients to realize that we doctors are humans and that we appreciate what they might do to help, such as bringing notes and questions to their appointments, arriving on time for appointments — maybe even early to complete paperwork — and doing whatever possible to build a personal connection. Just asking "How are you doing?" can mean a lot. This just happened to me as I was making rounds at the hospital, I was examining a newborn baby and talking to the mom about her newborn when the mom suddenly asked me how my day was going. That simple act of kindness made me feel so grateful.

It also helps us when our patients and their families become involved and aware, not afraid to ask questions and tell us details that might help us understand and treat what's going on. Remember, emotional and lifestyle details — a sick relative, pressures about work, relationships at home, or finances — can significantly affect one's health. So, try to be a partner to your doctor. You don't have to be a best friend, but your support is so important to us.

And it's not just doctors

I see a lot of parents in my practice who also are feeling burned out and displaying those same symptoms. COVID has definitely put more pressure on parents, especially those with school children needing to be guided and taught at home. And post-partum moms tended to be even more isolated during COVID, so it's a condition that so many can relate to.

I think just about anyone can relate to burnout these days. The reality is we all have had much more to cope with, in our work, in our daily lives. In addition to the AMA starting to roll out programs for doctors, I've found a couple of podcasts that are helpful. One is called "The Burnout Doctor Podcast," by Dr. Jessica Louie.[15] A pharmacist who experienced her own burnout and recovery, Dr. Louie addresses healthcare workers across the board — doctors, nurses, and pharmacists — telling stories and giving great solutions.

What the AMA suggests, and I believe it to be true for everyone, is that support is crucial. It does seem like a no-brainer, but it's important to get support from your family and friends, as well as from your colleagues.

My family was amazing. When I look back, I am reminded of how strong that support was. I mean, at first, they were kind of outraged with that label of "disruptive physician," just as I was. They realized I was facing a challenge to my core. And just as I did — maybe even before — they began to realize that I needed that break, they were concerned for me, and their care and support were phenomenal.

My colleagues also were so wonderful and supportive. Many of them don't know the extent of what I went through, exactly, but when I came back, they welcomed me with open arms. Some didn't seem to know what to say, so they said very little, but I felt the support and the friendship from my colleagues.

The truth is we have all been in a fight-or-flight mode, survival mode, and having that constant pressure, stress, and worry not only wears you down, but it's also terrible for your health. And when you are in charge, as a parent, a doctor, a nurse, or any healthcare worker, you are always functioning at a

---

[15] https://drjessicalouie.com/

high level, all your neurotransmitters, hormones and chemicals are at capacity collapse and burnout will follow.

Because that's the role you have taken on: protector. You promised to protect, and you promised to help. That's a physician's promise. It's a nurse's promise, and it's a parent's promise. You just keep going and going. Then when you hit the aftermath, you inevitably fall into fatigue, and everything comes to a crash. That's how my staff and I felt, and I still sometimes feel like I'm falling.

From break down to breakthrough

Yes, what's happening in my profession is also happening throughout our society. And not just with adults. The rise in teen suicide attempts and deaths is heartbreaking. There has been an increase of people, young and older, with seasonal depression.

In our practice, we have been seeing an increase in mothers with post-partum depression. A study done in 2021 at Harvard[16] looked at 6,894 post-partum women and found elevated levels of depression and anxiety (31%) and loneliness (53%), and 43% reported PTSD in relation to COVID, even though only 2% had actually had it. The study authors had a theory that being home so much exposed new mothers to excessive media covering the pandemic, which might have raised their anxiety levels, and they are depressed because they are concerned, on top of everything else.

Since this experience with burnout has been so widespread, my hope is that there will no longer be shame around it, that people can ask for help and love and support and find the resources and incredible tools they need.

What does it take to go from breakdown through breakthrough? It requires you to be awake and aware from birth all the way through your life. Next, we'll look at what that means.

---

[16] https://www.hsph.harvard.edu/news/press-releases/pregnant-postpartum-covid19-post-traumatic-stress/

"The reality is: there will always be more work. From our jobs and owning businesses, to being a manager of our families and our homes – there will always be more work. It never goes away. We never escape from the responsibilities that life presents us. But one of our main responsibilities should be ourselves, after all, there's only one of us anyway."

——Vanessa Autrey,
The Art of Balancing Burnout

Chapter 3

DARE TO BE AWARE

**Learn how to observe your health,
trust your instincts, and take action.
"Awareness is the first step of healing."**

— Dean Ornish,
author of *Undo It: How Simple Lifestyle Changes
Can Reverse Most Chronic Diseases*

**"To successfully open the door to heightened awareness,
we must open it inward."**

— Wayne Dyer

Attention, please

There's a term I use to describe the awareness and responsibility I'm asking you to embrace around your health and happiness: I call it "medical intuition." Intuition means the ability to understand something immediately, without the need for conscious reasoning.

Medical intuition means medical awareness, awareness of your own body and your own health, and your physical and emotional health. Trusting your intuition means you might have an inkling that something is happening, and you pay attention and take responsibility for acting, for doing something for yourself.

So, how does someone develop medical awareness and use it to their advantage? The key is observation.

Medical alignment and the art of observation

Every morning, when I wake up and even before getting out of bed, I do a self-check. Later I will teach you an energizing and illuminating Body Scan, but first, let me show you a simple self-check.

When you wake up in the morning, and while you are still lying down (and no kids or partners are relying on you for a few minutes), just ask yourself – *How do I feel?* Maybe you feel awesome. Ask yourself why: Did you have a great night's sleep? Was the day before active and fulfilling? Were your meals complete and rejuvenating? Can you take some deep, long breaths, and feel excited about your day?

And maybe you discover the opposite: Do you feel groggy and uninspired by the day ahead of you? The first thing to look at is your sleep: Did you wake up several times, and maybe have a hard time going back to sleep? Is your body sore and stiff because of the exercise you did yesterday? Did you just get a COVID booster? What did you eat? What did you drink? How was your day at work?

As I recounted for you in the introduction, I get migraine headaches — much less frequently than I used to, but occasionally I still do, and when I do, I do a self-check. If I find myself feeling miserable, I think about my day, the day before. I might recognize that I had an extremely busy day at the office, as I often do, and it was extremely challenging. And I had a conflict with somebody who is important to me, and I did not have a good night's sleep. Maybe I drank a little too much wine and skipped lunch because I was so busy. I might even feel a migraine coming on.

The opposite of medical awareness = medical misalignment

All of these internal and environmental elements can add up to what I call "misalignment." And the number one cause for misalignment is stress. So much of the time, especially if we don't recognize we are stressed, we will manifest it physically. We might try medication after medication and might feel like we are drowning in a vicious cycle. And this is when you ask yourself – *What is going on in my life? Why am I feeling this way?* Do your self-check and look for reasons.

If you don't identify the reasons, that's okay, too. But be aware of how you slept, and how you feel emotionally. Become conscious of your breathing; is it shallow? Be aware of what you drank last night, and what you ate yesterday. Ask yourself how active you are, what kind of people came into your life, and what kind of interactions you had.

This is the first step toward medical alignment: observation.

If you can connect what's happening in your body, what you are feeling in your muscles, your gut, your head, with what is happening with your emotions and your mind, you are coming closer to mind/body connection and balance. You are taking steps toward self-awareness and alignment. Medical misalignment occurs when you do not have the awareness that what's going on in your physical body is connected to your emotional and mental state.

> **"It's your road and yours alone.**
> **others may walk it with you,**
> **but no one can walk it for you."**

> — Rumi

PART 2

Chapter 4

THE BODY SCAN

**It's the first step to becoming aware of what's going on in
your body and your mind.**

*I*n his book *The Power of Now,* spiritual leader Eckhart Tolle writes about the power of a type of body scan, which he calls Inner Body Awareness meditation. At the age of 30, Tolle found himself at a rock bottom of anxiety and depression that led him to an epiphany and caused a remarkable turnabout. He was in a state of ecstasy and peace for five months, re-entered the world, and began using his education from the London and Cambridge universities to share his awakening with the world. He writes that using this body scan allows you to be deeply aware of the present moment and that regular practice will impart energy and sustained well-being, and possibly help ease pain, depression, and anxiety.

Here is a body scan I use with many of my patients and their parents. It only takes about 15 minutes. You can also go to my website and listen to a recording in which I walk you through it.

BODY SCAN MEDITATION #1

You can find a recording of me speaking this meditation at <u>www.drlamiakatbi.com</u> and listen, or record yourself speaking it, then play back.

- OK, I'm going to invite you to sit with your back straight if you can. Relax your shoulders, and I want you to just breathe naturally for now.

- Now, I invite you to close your eyes, or just relax, whatever you feel like. We want to start with breathing, just breathe naturally. We're going to breathe in through the nose. And exhale through the nose. Take a couple of breaths. Just like that.

- Again, pay attention to your shoulders. Make sure they're relaxed.

- If your legs are crossed, maybe consider not crossing them.

- And make sure that your eyes are soft. Relax your eyes.

- Now I'm going to ask you to think about last night. How did you sleep? What time did you go to bed? Was it what you wanted? Did you stay up late? Did you watch lots of television? Are you working? Do you feel like you slept?

- When you woke up this morning, did you feel refreshed? Or did you think, *I really wish I had slept longer?* Or, *I wish I had gone to bed earlier.* It is okay. Just breathe.

- Okay, now, I want to take you into your day yesterday. Did you have a good day? Did you have fun? Did you write? Did you do things that were relaxing to you? Productive?

- Did you have three meals or two? Did you make good choices when you ate? How you ate? Did you look at your food?

- I wonder if you watched TV while you were eating? Or were you mindful about how and where you ate? Did you eat alone? Or with family or friends?

- How do you feel about how much water you drank yesterday? Did you perhaps drink enough or not enough? What do you think? I want you to think about it. Do you think maybe you will make a more conscious decision to drink more water today or tomorrow? I wonder if you know how many ounces you need to drink every day.

- I wonder how much caffeine you had yesterday. And if you know this is right for you or maybe too much or maybe just enough. And that's okay. I'm just wondering.

- Did you have a conversation with somebody you're uncomfortable talking to? Did you have a difficult conversation recently? With anyone? How did you handle it? How did that make you feel? Angry? Happy? Relieved? Resentful. These are all emotions. And they are all okay to feel and it's okay to just let go of them.

- Now, I would like you to think about a sunny place, maybe it's a beach, maybe it's a mountain. Maybe it's a summer day. Maybe it's just somewhere near your house. Go for a walk. And listen to the ocean. The waves, feel the breeze, the warmth of the sun, on your skin, and breathe it in.

- Feel the love of nature, on your skin, on your hair, in your heart, in your gut. You go home. And now it's time to say to yourself, I am going to sleep. I did my physical activity by walking. I ate, and I took care of myself. And I feel good. I want you to feel good about your day.

- Now, we are going to end this brief exercise with breathing. We're going to inhale, take a normal breath. Breathe in and breathe out.

- We're going to do that another time. Breathe in. Breathe out, with a normal cadence. Now, I'm going to invite you to breathe in for five. I'm going to do the counting: 1, 2, 3, 4, 5. Pause at the top of the breath, then exhale through your nose. 1, 2, 3, 4, 5.

- We'll do it again. Inhale through your nose. 1, 2, 3, 4, 5. Pause at the top. Exhale for 1, 2, 3, 4, 5 one more time. Inhale through your nose. 1, 2, 3, 4, 5. Pause at the top. Exhale 1, 2, 3, 4, 5.

- Now we're going to breathe normally again. And I want you to scan your body. How do you feel? Your shoulders, your eyes, your hips, your hands, your thighs, your legs, your feet. I'm going to invite you to start to wiggle your fingers and your toes. If you need to move your head from side to side or slightly slowly and then very gently open your eyes come back to the present moment.

BODY SCAN MEDITATION #2

Another, simpler progressive relaxation is one from a book called *The PTSD Workbook*. In this technique, you focus on slowly tensing and then relaxing the muscles in your body. I'm a believer in presenting information in many different ways, so you have options here. If you want to read this exercise, then lie or sit down and do it, go for it. If you prefer to listen to me talk you through it, go to this link **www.drlamiakatbi.com** here you'll find a recording of my voice taking you through this progressive relaxation. You choose.

Progressive muscle relaxation practice

This sequence takes you from your head through your neck, shoulders, arms and hands, chest, back, stomach, hips, legs, and feet. Each of these steps is the tensing part; after tensing, you will release or relax those muscles. If you make yourself a recording of this exercise, be sure to allow enough time for each exercise — 5 to 7 seconds to tense and 20 to 30 seconds to release and not rush. Do two repetitions of each step. You can also start at your toes and work up if you like.

- Wrinkle your forehead.
- Squint your eyes tightly.
- Open your mouth wide.
- Push your tongue against the roof of your mouth.
- Clench your jaw tightly.
- Push your head back.
- Push your head forward to touch your chest.
- Roll your head to your right shoulder.
- Roll your head to your left shoulder.
- Shrug your shoulders up as if to touch your ear.
- Shrug your right shoulder up as if to touch your ear.

- Shrug your left shoulder up as if to touch your ear.
- Hold your arms out and make a fist with your hands.
- One side at a time, push your hand down to the surface where you are practicing.
- One side at a time, make a fist, bend your arm at the elbow, and tighten your arm while holding the fist.
- Take a deep breath and hold.
- Tighten your chest muscles.
- Arch your back.
- Tighten your abdominal area.
- Push your ab muscles out.
- Pull your ab muscles in.
- Tighten your hips, your glutes.
- Push the heels of your feet into the surface where you are practicing.
- Tighten the leg muscles below your knees.
- Curl your toes under as if to touch the bottoms of your feet.
- Flex your toes up as if to touch your knees.
- Relax and breathe softly for a few moments.

Adapted from: *The PTSD Workbook: Simple, Effective Techniques for Overcoming Traumatic Stress Symptoms*, by Mary Beth Williams

BODY SCAN MEDITATION #3

The UCLA Mindfulness Research Center offers many meditations on its website; here is a body scan meditation led by Director of Mindfulness Education, Diana Winston.

https://www.outofstress.com/inner-body-meditation/

Step 1: Feel the weight of your body

- Lie down comfortably on your bed, on your back or belly as per your preference.

- Close your eyes and feel the entire weight of your body being supported by your bed.

- Feel the parts of your body that are in contact with the surface of the bed.

- Realize that you need not make any effort to support your body. So completely let go and let the entire weight of your body sink into your bed.

- If you find this hard here's a simple visualization you can do: Think of your body as light as a feather as you are freely floating through the air. You completely let go and allow yourself to glide slowly through the air.

As you visualize this in your mind, it will be a lot easier for you to let go.

Step 2: Bring your attention to your breath

- Slowly bring your attention to your breathing. Breathe in deeply and relax as you breathe out.

- As you breathe in, feel the cool air caressing the inner walls of your nostrils, as it enters your inner body. Feel the air entering your lungs through your windpipe and as you do this, feel your lungs expand. Hold your breath for a few seconds and feel this air inside your lungs. Realize that you are holding in pure life energy and that you are surrounded by it.

- Now breathe out and while doing so, feel your lungs deflate while also feeling the warmth of the air caressing the insides of your nostrils and upper lips as it glides out.

- Repeat this a few times.

- If your attention gets lost in your thoughts any time during this exercise, gently bring it back to "feeling." As you feel, part of your attention will be on the images that your mind produces and that is perfectly fine. The idea is to stay alert so you are not fully lost in these images and that a major part of your attention is always on the feeling.

After feeling your breath this way for roughly a minute or two, let's now start to feel some other parts of your body.

Step 3: Feel the soles of your feet

- Shift your attention to the soles of your feet. See if you can sense any sensations here. In most cases, it would be a light tingling sensation or a sensation of warmth. You can also sense mild aches at times. Spend a few seconds here.

- Slowly move your attention to your calf muscles, your knees and then to your thigh muscles followed by the muscles in and around your glutes and lower back.

- You can start with the left leg and move to the right or do both at the same time.

  Note: Your attention can be at multiple places within your body at the same time. For example, you can feel both your palms and soles of your feet at the same time, or you can keep your attention localized at a single point, like the palm of your right hand or the sole of your left foot.

Step 4: Feel your gut area

- Feel in and around your gut area. Often times when you are stressed, you tend to unconsciously clench this area, so if you find any tension in this area, let go and let it soften.

- Move your attention to your stomach/abdomen area and do the same. Feeling and relaxing your gut and stomach this way can help immensely in the digestion process and heal any related issues that you might have.

Step 5: Feel your heart area

- Slowly move your attention up to your chest area. Feel your heart beating and pumping life energy to all parts of your body. Realize that your heart has been beating non-stop since the beginning.

If you want, you can place a hand over your heart to feel the beats.

Step 6: Feel the palms of your hands

- Shift your attention now to your traps and shoulders, and then to your arms, elbows, forearms, wrists, and fingers. Feel the tip of your fingers and then the entire palm of your hands. See if you can sense the movement of energy in your palms.

Step 7: Feel your neck area

- Move your attention to the front and back of your neck and then onto your upper and lower back. Try to feel your spinal cord and the muscles surrounding it. As you do this, once again feel the entire weight of your back resting against the bed.

Step 8: Feel your head area

- Bring your attention to the top of your head, spend a few seconds and see if you feel any sensations here. There is a high likelihood that you might feel a tingling sensation. If you don't feel any sensation, do not worry. Just relax this area.

- Now move your attention to the back of your head and feel its entire weight lying on the pillow. If you find any tightness in this area, which is highly possible, gently let go and relax.

- Take your attention to the sides of your head, your forehead, and then onto your facial muscles, eyes, lips, and the inside of your mouth. Spend a few seconds in each of these areas and see if you feel any sensations and consciously relax these areas.

Step 9: Feel your entire body

- Now let your attention run freely within your body. Shift your attention anywhere you feel an ache, tingling, or tightness and relax these areas.

- Before you finish this exercise, and in most cases, when you are midway, you should be already deep asleep.

Adapted from *Inner Body Meditation Technique to Experience Deep ....* *https://www.outofstress.com/inner-body-meditation/*

The benefits of meditation

I've spoken about my time at the Professional Renewal Center, and how fortunate I feel that I was to be able to go there for an extended amount of time and learn certain tools that helped me heal and find my way back to health and happiness. Meditation is one of those tools. Before I went to the Center, I dabbled, but the regular practice is so valuable in allowing your body to relax, and to become aware of what's happening in your body and your life, to become aware of your emotional and physical being. There are many other benefits, too:

1. **Calm** – By doing the body scan meditation — any meditation really — you will notice that you feel calmer than before, that you wake up without anxiety. You might also notice that your thought becomes clearer, that you can calmly think about something for a long time, without reacting to stimuli and jumping around in your mind. Your racing thoughts slow down.

2. **Relaxation** – Meditation will help you relax your body and help you feel present and mindful. The breathing, the progressive body relaxation, the encouragement to become aware of your body and emotions, and what is happening inside you, will all culminate in deep relaxation. You can also do a body scan or relaxation mediation as a sleep tool.

3. **Emotional intelligence** – Because you are calming your racing mind, you might become more intuitive and empathetic. You can listen to others and hear their needs without reacting impulsively; you can be more attentive to your own needs, too.

4. **Stress reduction** – A regular practice of meditation can reduce stress by diverting your body's priorities from the "fight or flight" mechanism to a calm, healing state, and opens you up to deep healing.

Here's a quick and easy practice that can be done anytime. I love it because my son told me how it helped him during test anxiety and whenever he feels uneasy:

1.   Name five things you can see
2.   Four things you can feel
3.   Three things you can hear
4.   Two things you taste or smell
5.   And one positive thought.

Obviously, you can modify it the way you want. but it is such a powerful exercise to disrupt your thoughts and to bring you to the present moment.

The late Louise Hay taught a body scan during which she would invite listeners to let go of harmful patterns in their lives. She started by asking them to tense the whole body, making it tighter and tighter like a tight, tight ball, then to take a deep, deep inhale and fill up like a big balloon, then exhale completely. Taking another deep breath, and as you exhale, picture yourself in a beautiful place, a place you love, surrounded by people, animals, plants, whatever is meaningful and safe to you. Stay in this place and feel your body relax more and more deeply until you are ready to come back into the world.

I have found teachers such as Louise Hay, Wayne Dyer, Eckhart Tolle, Thich Nhat Hanh, who passed away just this year, all share teaching points, and one is awareness; another is the breath.

Trust your self

When you use your medical awareness, your medical intuition — for yourself or for your child, by the way — you can sense when something is off. I cannot emphasize this enough, and I see it again and again in my practice: If a parent tells me something is going on, I trust them, because they know their child and most parents are more in tune with their child's health than they are their own. Why? Because their children are most important to them and they are responsible for their children's health and happiness, while, at the same time, parents sometimes tend to ignore their health.

It always fascinates me. We mothers get to know our children as we carry them for nine months, and then we get to see them as newborns and witness that magic, that miracle of life. During my first pregnancy, I was feeling uptight and nervous as many first-time parents do. You want to be perfect, dont want to make mistakes or mess up take as many photos as you possibly can, and it puts a lot of pressure on both of you: the firstborn child and the parents. If the parents already have their own emotional, mental and physical struggles , those issues will somehow make presence and affect the children, especially the first born.

And of course, by the time I had my third child I was much more relaxed, although I see parents often doing what I'm sure I did, and that's telling the older siblings what a good big sister or brother they will be. They are three or four years old! More pressure, to be Mommy's or Daddy's helper, and it's another thing to look at when you look at the trajectory of your life, and your children's lives. And while we mothers tend to feel responsible for everything that happens to our children, sometimes it's just not practical.

I'm inviting you to become responsible for *your* own health and happiness.

Using Dr. Google

As I mentioned before, we have a wonderful tool available to us on the internet. It's just that you have to be careful when you search, because if you don't have a medical background and you go on "Dr. Google," or one of the many mom's groups on social media — there are so many of them now — you just have to be careful how to read and how to interpret the information you're reading. If you don't have a medical background, or experience reading studies and journals and articles, you are going to jump to the worst-case scenario and be convinced you have cancer.

For instance, I had a patient whose diagnosis was hand, foot, and mouth disease, which is common in children. I searched for some pictures to show the parents. And seriously, they show you the worst possible cases, instead of transitioning from the most common to the most serious. You'd think the child was bleeding from head to toe.

A dad brought his toddler son to the office complaining of a couple of bruises on his legs, the bruises were impressive in size. The toddler was active, but there was no bruising anywhere else on his body. The father told me he had searched the Internet for answers and couldn't sleep that night. I asked him, "What did Dr. Google say?"

He sighed and said, "Dr. Katbi, Dr. Google killed my son five times last night."

So when you search for stuff, you have to be careful. If something is bothering you, you search and you get scared while reading, you need to stop and tell yourself – *that's enough, I need to reach out to my healthcare provider.* And that's it, remember that Dr. Google really means you are self-diagnosing and go get yourself some professional help.

Here's another example of the power of social media. I had a patient, a 13-year-old boy who came in with his mother and told me he had concerns about ADHD (attention deficit hyperactivity disorder). We went over the criteria and discussed testing, and I came back to him and said, "You know, you do have some components of ADHD. And he immediately said, "I knew it!" When I asked him how he knew it, he said, "I watched TikTok. There is a person on TikTok spreading awareness about ADHD."

So, this was someone who probably has been diagnosed with ADHD, but other than that has no qualifications or background that would make it appropriate for them to be diagnosing anyone. As we know kids are following influencers on social media, and my fear is that without proper medical management they might seek out street drugs and self-medicate. If TikTok leads them to see a doctor, great. Spreading awareness is great, but the next step has to be medical consultation and care.

This is true for all other media platforms. We need to be curious about the information presented to us and learn more about it before we make it factual.

Responsibility vs. guilt

Once you start taking responsibility for your own health and well-being, you are bound to make a mistake occasionally. Everyone does. It could be a decision you made, and an action you took — or didn't take — something you procrastinated about.

Instead of fretting about it, going down that rabbit hole of feeling guilty and blaming yourself, just stop. Admit your responsibility, admit your mistake, and act upon it. Just take the next step. Apologize if it is appropriate, if you inadvertently hurt someone else, and move on.

I still find a lot of people who are in denial about their health, or certain diseases such as heart disease, obesity, and eating disorders, addiction, and even sexual health issues. They feel guilty, but they don't want to take responsibility. It's so interesting to me that they feel guilty but won't admit their failure. They made some bad decisions but won't take that responsibility, and instead get bogged down by the guilt.

For decades we doctors have been talking about healthy diets and exercise. We barely even touch on the other Pillars of Sleep, Breathing, and Emotional Health, because so many people have no awareness, even of the most widely known factors that affect one's health. Maybe it's harsh to use the word "ignorance," but that's exactly what it is. Ignorance.

At the same time, how can we call people/ourselves ignorant if we do not have knowledge or awareness of the lack of it? I will take the first bullet here and admit that I was ignorant of my own health and my own well-being. I ignored my basic needs of allowing myself to be happy and to practice self-care.

It IS a lack of awareness, a lack of education. Even now, with such easy access to information through browsing online, you may get different information. This information can be false or unverified, so we need to be very careful about how we use the information we get through the internet. That's why I recommend following reputable sites, such as the CDC, AAP, AMA, WebMD, and websites associated with major medical schools and health institutions such as Harvard Health and Johns Hopkins. We need to do our homework before we can use those resources, especially when it comes to our own health and wellness. We also need to adapt and change as things evolve and change. Unless we have the foundation and awareness of how to interpret the information we get, we might do more harm than good.

That's why I educate/guide the parents in my practice. I believe home is the first and most important school for children. Kids observe and absorb at such a young age. Our job as parents is to become the role model we wish our parents were for us.

Chapter 5

THE FIVE-PILLAR BODY SCAN QUIZ

The Inner Body Awareness Meditation you have learned, either by listening to my audio, or to any other type of body scan meditation, is primarily to increase your medical intuition and awareness, and also to relax and energize you. Perhaps you read my words and repeat them to yourself as you do an inner scan; maybe you use it to relax yourself to sleep.

Now it's time to do some healing work, work that will examine where you stand in terms of the concept I introduced to you previously: **The Five Pillars of Optimal Health.** Here they are again:

Sleep
Emotional Health
Mindful Eating
Intentional Breath
Physical Activity

In this directed **body scan quiz,** I'm going to ask questions to bring your awareness to each of the pillars, give you some suggestions of ways to keep track of your progress, then go into detail about each, why they are so important, and how to improve on the pillars that need strengthening. I encourage you to use a journal to record your answers and your thoughts – more about that later.

1. **Sleep** I want you to think about how you sleep.

   - *Do* you sleep? Do you sleep well?

   - How many hours of sleep do you get each night? Do you get 7 to 8 hours? Five?

   - How many hours do you think you need each night?

   - What time do you go to bed?

   - Do you have a hard time falling asleep? Do you wake up in the middle of the night and have trouble going back to sleep?

   - Is your phone next to you? Do you check social media or browse the web?

   - Do you listen to music?

   - Do you have a TV in your bedroom? Do you watch TV before bed?

   - Do you dream?

   - Do you drink coffee before going to bed? Do you drink alcohol before going to bed?

   - Do you wake up to an alarm clock?

   - What is the room temperature in your room? What is ideal?

   - How dark is your room at night?

   - What is your bedtime routine and ritual?

2. **Emotional Health** Examine your relationships and feelings.

   - Do you feel happy? Sad?

   - How do you take care of yourself on that level?

   - When you look at yourself in the mirror, do you see a good person? A beautiful person? Or otherwise?

   - Do you talk to friends and family often?

   - Do you have a healthy relationship with your mother and father? Your siblings? Your children?

- Do you have a healthy romantic relationship?
- Do you cry often, or feel anxious often?
- What do you do to calm yourself when you are stressed?
- Do you feel depressed? Do you take any medications for depression or anxiety?
- Are you hard on yourself? Do you talk to yourself kindly? Do you forgive yourself for your mistakes? Do you punish yourself? Do you feel compassion toward yourself?

3. **Mindful Eating** I want you to think about how you eat.
   - How do you feel about the way you eat?
   - Do you feel you are a healthy eater? And what is a healthy diet?
   - Do you follow a strict diet?
   - Do you eat breakfast, lunch, and dinner?
   - Do you ever do intermittent fasting? Do you feel skipping meals is a good thing for you?
   - Do you drink lots of water? Do you know how much water your body needs every day? Do you drink caffeine? Sugary drinks? Alcohol?
   - Do you vape/ smoke?
   - Are you eating a lot of processed food, such as boxed or frozen dinners, chips, or candy?
   - Do you like how your body looks? Are you trying to lose weight?
   - Do you watch TV or go on social media while eating dinner?
   - Do you chew your food, and eat fast or slow?
   - Is how your food looks important to you?
   - Do you eat dinner as a family?
   - Do you stop eating when you feel full?
   - Do you snack while watching TV?

4. **Intentional Breath** Become aware of your breath.

   - How do you breathe? Are you curious about the way you breathe?
   - Do you breathe shallowly? Deeply?
   - Do you breathe mostly through your mouth, or through your nose?
   - When you're challenged with a situation, do you feel you're holding your breath?
   - Are you familiar with different types of breathing?
   - Do you practice any mindful breathing?
   - Do you use your breath intentionally every day?
   - Do you get panicky sometimes?
   - What do you do to stay grounded?
   - Are you aware of abdominal breathing vs chest breathing?
   - Do you take slow inhales and exhales?
   - Do you thank yourself for your breath every morning?
   - Are you concerned about your breathing while you're asleep? Sleep apnea?

5. **Physical Activity** Let's examine your physical body.

   - What is your level of fitness?
   - Do you move your body daily? How active are you on daily basis?
   - Do you work out at all? Every day? Three to four times a week?
   - Do you avoid walking distances? Climbing? Running?
   - After you work out strenuously, do you rest? Do you take supplements, and/or protein shakes?
   - Do you go to a gym? Swim? Ride a bike? Hike in nature?
   - Do you have any injuries that inhibit your ability to be active? If so, what are you doing about them?

- Do you like working out alone, with a group?
- Do you work out in the morning, midday, or evening?
- Do you stretch before or after your workout?
- Do you combine strength training with cardio?

When I lead someone through this body scan and I can see them, whether in person or on Zoom, I watch them, I notice when they smile, when they tense up, and when something I say has hit them. See if you can notice that about yourself.

Chapter 6

TOOLS FOR AWARENESS: JOURNALS AND APPS

**Note where you are now and
keep track of your progress**

**"Writing in a journal each day allows you to direct your
focus to what you accomplished, what you're grateful for,
and what you're committed to doing better tomorrow.
Thus, you more deeply enjoy your journey each day."**

— Hal Elrod, author, *The Miracle Morning*

**"Write what disturbs you, what you fear, what you have
not been willing to speak about.
Be willing to be split open."**

— Natalie Goldberg

Write it down

I have been journaling off and on for as long as I can remember, mostly when I feel sad and lonely, when I feel I need to let something out that is bothering me, but don't know how to express it. I always feel better after writing; for me writing is cathartic. I actually enjoy it when I go back and read something I wrote years ago. It is grounding to know the progress I have made, the then and the now are so powerful and a beautiful reminder of how our lives evolve.

My daughter gave me a beautiful journal for Christmas one year. She knows me so well. I believe in writing in a journal, each day if possible. But you don't have to be perfect; in fact, I encourage the opposite of perfect. Just write.

There are many different ways to journal; some people use an At-A-Glance planner, even just a regular calendar. And there are many different motivations. I've noticed that I write in my diary much more when I'm sad than when I'm happy. Just as sometimes it's easier to write a song about being heartbroken than being in love. It's as if I don't have as much need to write when I'm happy; but it's still important to get those thoughts down, so you can look back at them.

For our purposes here, you can use your journal to write down the answers to the body scan quiz, you can write your thoughts about how you are doing in each of the **Five Pillars of Optimal Health,** how you would like to improve, what your frustrations and obstacles might be, and what can you do to be successful in your health journey.

You can start with a blank journal, and fill it up as you go, with quizzes, inspirations, fears, triumphs, wishes, and wins. Or, you can get a journal with prompts, such as The Five-Minute Journal, which gives you prompts, challenges, ideas, and inspiration. It's from Intelligent Change Products, about $30, and will last you six months if you write every day. I like it because it comes with a nice linen cover (a choice of six colors) and just feels good to hold.

There are many apps you can use to keep track of your progress and build healthy habits. *Fabulous: Self Care* was created at Duke University and uses behavioral science to help you make healthful lifestyle changes. It was named the Best Self-Care app by Apple and works with Android too; the basic subscription is free and there are several upgrades. It's bright and fun, and I don't know about you, but I love a good quiz.

Whatever moves you most, the goal is becoming aware, responsible, and involved in your own health and happiness.

Developing awareness 101

My mornings are sacred to me – that's when I meditate, express gratitude, journal, and get grounded for the day ahead. That is when many self-help coaches — Louise Hay, Jay Shetty, Julia Cameron, Gabby Bernstein, and Hal Elrod, among many others — suggest you carve out time for yourself and create a morning routine.

Morning time is when I believe you are most connected with your inner self; the day hasn't crept in and infiltrated your mind yet. So, before you get dressed — you can stay in bed, sit at the edge of your bed, or even get your morning cup of Joe — connect to your inner self. You can call it meditation, it's a wonderful time of day to meditate, but you don't even have to call it that, just so you take time to go deep, be mindful of who you are and where you are, what progress you have been making. Start to be aware of what's around you, where you are today, and how you are feeling at that moment.

Sometimes, on my day off, I give it 30 minutes, but five or ten minutes is my go-to most workdays, which is plenty. I don't turn on the news in the morning; I stopped listening to the news years ago. I wake up early, typically between 5 and 5:30 a.m. to give me enough time to feel centered, grounded, and ready for the day ahead. I do not use an alarm clock; I've found I don't need it.

When I wake up, I do check my phone to make sure I didn't miss any calls from the hospital or the service, but I avoid checking any social media or emails. I make my bed, I make my coffee, then I sit in one of my favorite spots at home — it depends on what season we are in — and just sit still.

I scan my body and depending on how I feel, I choose what type of breathing exercise or meditation I will do. Sometimes silence is all I need, and other times I listen to guided meditation or breathing.

I journal most days — I journal more when I feel conflicted or triggered by a thought or an event. The last thing I do when I have extra time is listen to motivational speakers on YouTube, again such as Jay Shetty, Wayne Dyer, The Power of Positivity, The Law of Attraction, Oprah Winfrey and Steve Harvey, to name just a few. It took me years of practice to get to where I am today and I still struggle to focus sometimes. And I'm not one to keep the television on in the background; I think it all goes into your subconsciousness. And it's a distraction, even when we believe otherwise.

Other ways to develop awareness include nature walks. Any mindful physical activity, especially walking outdoors in nature, can improve health. Many studies have found that nature walks, especially with a group, can increase resilience and reduce mental stress and anxiety. [17] Of course, the physical act of walking brings blood to the brain, allows concentration, and is good for the heart, but there's something about getting your feet on the ground, seeing trees and plants, greenery, and even hugging a tree (which I do actually). These same studies have found that the amount of foliage surrounding a home influences the stress levels of its occupants, including children.

And while I don't follow a specific religion, I find prayer, using your faith, is absolutely powerful to make you more aware of your life and your goals. If you belong to a congregation, you can invite them to share your journey; you might even find a support group to help you. To me, prayer is asking, and meditation is listening to the answers.

The importance of a safe place

If you have gotten this far, you are already building your awareness, and with it your sense of worthiness. You are opening up and actually doing the work. It's not easy to open those wounds.

---

[17] https://www.ncbi.nlm.nih.gov/pmc/articles/PMC6466337/ Growing Resilience through Interaction with Nature:

That's why you have to do it in a safe environment. In retrospect, I realize how lucky I was to be sent to PRC. When I was in the middle of it, I kept thinking about how "they" sent me there and I blamed them, I blamed myself, I blamed the world. But I was lucky to be there, I feel I was given a second chance. Yes, I was asked to go and had to do the work, but I was surrounded by professionals, and I continued the work even after I left, with therapists and trusted friends and family.

I'm not saying you have to go to Lawrence, Kansas to get results. Find a family member, doctor, pastor, or a friend you can talk to. Finding the right therapist is extremely, extremely powerful. Even a podcast, listening to Brené Brown, Lewis Howes, Louise Hay, and Wayne Dyer can teach you awareness, and ease your anxiety. That's how I was introduced to lots of my mentors, by listening to YouTube motivational speeches and podcasts.

A patient of mine recently called me. She's 20 now, so she has aged out of my practice, but she wanted to make an appointment with me, just to talk. She had come to trust me as not only a doctor but also as a mentor. that was a powerful realization of the importance of having someone who can listen to you when you need it, and someone you can trust. Most importantly, someone who is there for you without any judgment. It's as if she recognized me as part of her village.

So find your village, connect with people who care about you and are there for you when you need them most. I personally have a beautiful village that includes many of my family members, my friends, and the professionals I go to when I need more help. You cannot do all this on your own. You need your village.

PART 3

THE FIVE PILLARS
OF A HEALTH ACTION PLAN

Your Path to Optimal Health

"To build a habit, you need to practice it. To be able to adhere to a practice you will need to:

- Make it easy; the most effective way of learning is practice, not planning
- Focus on taking action, not being in motion
- Repetition is what leads to the habit becoming automatic

The amount of time you have been performing a habit is not as important as the number of times you have performed it..."

– James Clear, *Atomic Habits*

Pillar #1

SLEEP

**"Sleep is the golden chain that ties health and
our bodies together."**

— Thomas Dekker,
American actor

"Sleep is the best meditation."

— Dalai Lama

> Refer to page 54 for your sleep
> quiz questions and answers.

The need for sleep

I didn't understand the importance of sleep and how it affects all areas
of our health until a few years ago. I still have guilty feelings about
an incident that happened when I was a senior resident at the University of
Chicago. One night I was on call, which again means you spend your night
in the hospital taking care of sick patients and new admissions through the
emergency room. As a senior resident you are privileged to go to your on-call
room and sleep, and let the intern do the work first.

My intern was called to the emergency room with an admission, he did the initial history and physical exam, then tried to call me. He called and called, and I never answered him, and I never made it to the emergency room. In fact, I didn't wake up until the next morning, feeling panicked because I slept all night. The look on the intern's face told me how upset he was. Even though I apologized to him I felt so guilty then, and years later as well. I still feel uneasy when I think of that incident. I simply felt exhausted, but I didn't give myself permission to feel that way.

And it really opened my eyes to the importance of sleep, and how much it affects your mental health and ability to function. At the time, as I'm sure you can imagine, I felt like I had to be going, going, going, all the time. Because I wanted everything: I wanted to be married, I wanted to be a physician, I wanted to come to the United States, I wanted to have children. So I just kept pushing myself. And I was exhausted. That was the first time my lack of sleep had an impact on someone else, though. So, I learned that lesson. Sort of.

Being a physician means your sleep is interrupted and disrupted for most of your life. You are always anticipating being paged (a previous way of communication), or called or getting text messages from your office, patients, hospital, and answering service. It becomes second nature to you to be always on the lookout, and this means you are constantly in "fight-or-flight" mode. You dread those calls and messages, yet you're always on the lookout.

Because of that, many physicians sleep very poorly; they keep going because that is the only thing they know until one day it catches up with them. In my case, I know for a fact that my poor sleep affected my health negatively. Of course, I'm not saying that was the cause of my health issues, but I'm positive it played a major role in my illness, and in the way I reacted and interacted with people around me.

Sleep deprivation is not exclusive to health care workers

Most Americans do not get the sleep they need, and it's a big problem for our mental and physical health. The Centers for Disease Control estimates that 50 to 70 million adults have a chronic sleep disorder and that one in three adults gets less than seven hours of sleep a night.[18] Research associates not getting enough sleep with health conditions such as heart disease, asthma, high blood pressure, stroke, obesity, depression, diabetes, and even cancer.

Research reported by the National Health Institute even showed that a lack of sleep can impair abilities as much as getting drunk.[19] The study found that after 17 hours without sleep, our alertness is similar to the effects of a blood alcohol concentration of 0.05%, which <u>according to U.S. law</u> is considered "impaired" on the legally drunk scale, or even worse.

Research for the National Health and Aging Trends Study done at Harvard Medical School found that participants (who were all over 65) who reported sleeping fewer than five hours per night were twice as likely to develop dementia, and twice as likely to die, compared to those who slept six to eight hours per night.[20] And researchers in Europe (including France, the United Kingdom, the Netherlands, and Finland) examined data from almost 8,000 participants and found that consistently sleeping six hours or less at ages 50, 60, and 70 was associated with a 30% increase in dementia risk compared to a normal sleep duration of seven hours. [21]

Sleep is when you recharge, you heal, and your body rejuvenates and cleanses itself. When you don't get enough, or quality, sleep, maybe you will function okay today, but how about the next day and the day after that? There is no way you can go on day after day without sleep. It will affect your physical and mental health; we know you can actually get sick from not sleeping well, and it definitely can increase anxiety. Even anger.

You might find yourself getting shorter and shorter with your co-workers and your family. You overreact and might not even realize it. It's as if you revert to primitive coping methods, the fight or flight reaction, that you are using your

---

[18] https://www.cdc.gov/sleep/data_statistics.html

[19] https://www.ncbi.nlm.nih.gov/pmc/articles/PMC1739867/pdf/v057p00649.pdf

[20] https://www.aging-us.com/article/202591/text

[21] https://www.nature.com/articles/s41467-021-22354-2

amygdala — the part of your brain associated with strong emotions such as fear and anger — instead of your much more logical frontal cortex.

Sleep recommendations by age

Most people do not even know how much sleep they need. Sleep scientist Matthew Walker, PhD is the founder of the Center for Human Sleep Science and author of *Why We Sleep*. His specialty is describing how our sleep requirements change as we grow and age.

Fetuses get about 12 hours of REM sleep (rapid eye movement – the deep state of sleep characterized by fast brain activity) during the final 12 weeks of pregnancy, which builds neural pathways in the developing brain.

Newborn babies, of course, sleep 14 to 17 hours a day. We call it "Eat, sleep, repeat." But I like to start sleep training as early as possible; I recommend a nice warm bath followed by massage, dimming the lights, and maybe introducing some white noise (all of which apply to older children and adults, too). The room should be dark and quiet and cool, around the upper-60s in temperature.

Older Children need 10 to 11 hours of sleep each night, but their sleep is dominated by non-REM sleep (NREM) a stage characterized by slower brain wave activity, which Walker explains allows the brain to dispose of "trash," move memories into long-term storage and retain the most valuable associations.

Adolescents tend to stay up later and sleep later, which often doesn't sync with school start times; while they often are getting between 6 to 7 hours of sleep per night, the sleep tends to be disrupted; one NIH study Walker cites found that teens who adhere to parental-set bedtimes are more alert and less tired during the day. [22]

By the age of 18, our sleep needs decrease slightly. Adults need seven to nine hours of sleep, but as we age out of our 20s, sleep quality might deteriorate. The National Institute on Aging states that people over the age of 60 needing less sleep is a myth.

----

[22] https://pubmed.ncbi.nlm.nih.gov/21629368/

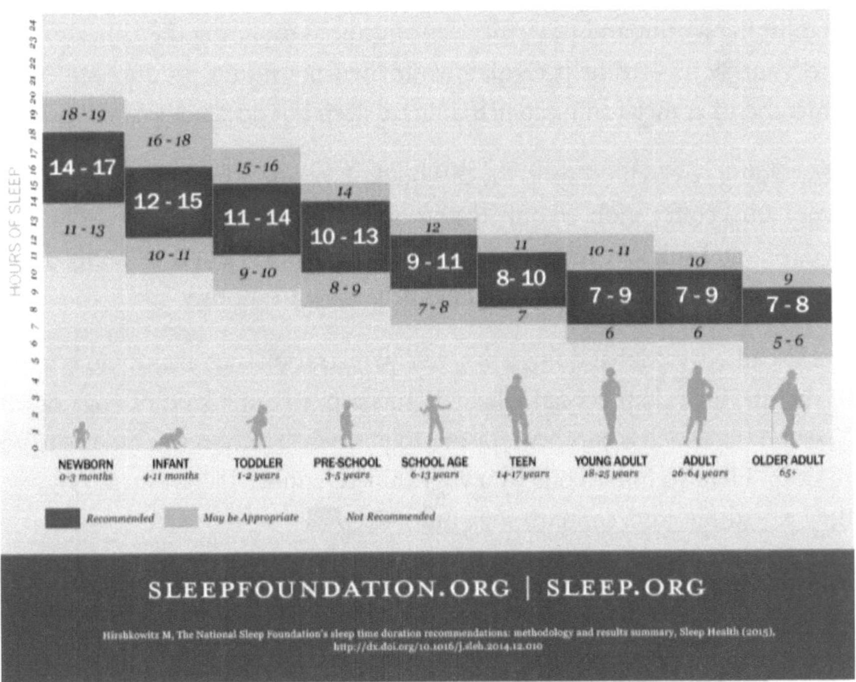

HOW TO GET THE SLEEP YOU NEED

The key to getting the amount and quality of sleep you need is to become aware of your **sleep hygiene.** Are you dimming the lights at night and avoiding screen time for at least one to two hours before bed? Going to bed at the same time each night, even on the weekends, is a big one, which most of us neglect.

Don't take your phone to bed, and don't have your TV in your bedroom. Take a nice warm shower before bed, and make sure your bedroom is cool, dark, and quiet. Try to go to sleep at the same time each night, even if it's the weekend; I like to say, "strive" to go to bed at the same time, but if you're busy, or sick, things will shift, and that's okay. You will find that your child's sleep training might shift, too, during the holidays or travel, don't cause yourself too much stress about it.

There also are supplements I recommend taking, such as magnesium, and some people like melatonin, although melatonin is a hormone our body produces to regulate our sleep cycles, and many experts do not recommend it as a supplement. Talk to your doctor before trying it: they might suggest establishing a calm and peaceful sleep routine – dimming the lights, easing into your sleep – to help regulate your own melatonin production. Also, remember that melatonin can help initiate sleep but does not maintain sleep.

After doing research on sleep for this book, I stopped drinking coffee after 1 p.m. I am a coffee snob, so only the strongest brew would do, and I drank it all day long. I still love my morning full-strength brew, but now I only drink one decaf coffee early afternoon. It has helped tremendously.

I've also discovered that doing a progressive relaxation such as any you learned in the previous chapters can relax you to sleep; so can a kind of yoga called Yoga Nidra, which is another type of progressive relaxation you can use to go to sleep. Here's a link to one by a yogi named Jennifer Piercy: https://www.doyogawithme.com/content/yoga-nidra-sleep

You also can use the Relaxing Breath at the end of this chapter.

SLEEP ACTION PLAN

Bestselling author Shawn Stevenson's 2016 book, *Sleep Smarter: 21 Essential Strategies to Sleep Your Way to a Better Body, Better Health and Better Success* outlines his personal discovery of the importance of sleep and the dangers of sleep deprivation. His background is in biology and kinesiology, and he is the founder of the Advanced Integrative Health Alliance. My coach Lewis Howes interviewed him for his podcast (if you like to listen to podcasts, check it out, below).[23]

Stevenson tells us that ultra-deep REM sleep is our most important stage of sleep because that's when your brain "converts your [daily] experiences

---

[23] https://lewishowes.com/podcast/shawn-stevenson-sleep/

into short-term memories, and eventually long-term memories. If you're not sleeping well, you miss most of that process."

Your quality of sleep affects your body as well, according to Stevenson: "A study published in the <u>Canadian Medical Association Journal</u> showed the impact of sleep on two groups of exercisers: Group A slept eight-plus hours a night, while Group B was sleep-deprived with around five hours of sleep per night. Group A lost far more weight and body fat than Group B, yet the only difference was the amount of sleep that they were getting."

Here are Shawn Stevenson's top 10 tips for getting the sleep you need:

1. **Get outside and get more sunlight** This will encourage the production of serotonin, a neurotransmitter that makes us feel good. It also converts into melatonin, the hormone that regulates our circadian rhythms, the sleep-wake cycles we go through each day. Nothing fancy, he says, just get outside, even if it's cold.

2. **Avoid screens close to bedtime** Another chemical in our brain is dopamine and it is related to seeking pleasure. "And guess how millions of us seek pleasure all day long? Through our screens — phones, computers, tablets, televisions — where there are always opportunities to read exciting articles, see hilarious cat videos, and connect with people we care about. It's like a slow drip of drugs, really!" says Stevenson. To avoid suppressing melatonin, avoid screens at least 60 to 90 minutes before bedtime.

3. **Cut back on caffeine** Research has found even six hours before bed can have a negative effect on sleep.

4. **Stay cool** "Your body goes through a process called thermal regulation every night to lower your core body temperature and create the ideal environment for deep sleep," according to Stevenson. Experts suggest keeping the thermostat between 62 and 68 degrees.

5. **Find the perfect bedtime** Studies show that anytime between 10 pm and 11 p.m., and, that it's important to be as consistent as possible. If it's not, focus on the other strategies even more.

6. **Black out your bedroom** "Photoreceptors [in our skin!] pick up information and send it to the brain to secrete more daytime hormones," says Stevenson. Your neighbor's porch light, streetlights outside, this unnatural light [has] been dubbed light pollution. Getting your room pitch black can keep that stuff out of your room. Be wary of internal lights too. An ugly alarm clock staring at you has the same effect. Or a nightlight!

7. **Train hard, but smart** A study was done with Appalachian State University breaking exercisers into three groups: Group A exercised at 7:00 a.m., Group B at 1:00 p.m., Group C 7:00 p.m. Group A spent up to 75% more time in deep anabolic sleep which is what you need to allow your body to rejuvenate each night.

8. **Go easy on the booze** Research shows that while drinking alcohol before bed might help you fall asleep faster, it might prevent you from staying asleep. Leave a few hours after your last drink before you hit the sack.

9. **Take the right supplements** Stevenson agrees that melatonin might not be for everyone and cites a study showing the supplement might interfere with your body's natural production. He suggests starting with chamomile or Kava.

10. **Get grounded** I've talked about the power of walking in nature. Stevenson is a believer that the earth is a powerful conductor of free electrons and protons, and that "when you get grounded which means getting your body connected to the earth's surface — inflammation goes down and your parasympathetic nervous system kicks on." This means your sympathetic system [the fight or flight response] gets switched off. "The conductive surfaces that do this," he says, "are anything from grass, dirt, soil, sand — even concrete is a little bit conductive." So kick off your shoes or gloves and get grounded for a while.

Next, we'll explore the second Pillar of Optimal Health: Emotional Health.

THE RELAXING BREATH

Don't forget the inner body scan meditations you have learned; these can help you drift off to sleep. Integrative physician Andrew Weil, MD, teaches a relaxing breath, AKA the 4-7-8 breath, that can help put you to sleep.

- Exhale completely through your mouth, making a *whoosh* sound.

- Close your mouth and inhale quietly through your nose to a mental count of **four**.

- Hold your breath for a count of **seven**.

- Exhale completely through your mouth, making a *whoosh* sound to a count of **eight**.

- This is one breath. Now inhale again and repeat the cycle three more times for a total of four breaths.

Do this in bed instead of counting sheep. It really works.

EMOTIONAL HEALTH

"Perfectionism is not the same thing as striving to be your best. Perfectionism is the belief that if we live perfectly, look perfect, and act perfect, we can minimize or avoid the pain of blame, judgment, and shame. It's a shield. It's a twenty-ton shield that we lug around thinking it will protect us when, in fact, it's the thing that's really preventing us from flight."

—Brené Brown, *The Gifts of Imperfection:*
Let Go of Who You Think You're Supposed to Be and Embrace
Who You Are

> Refer to page 54 for your emotional
> health quiz questions and answers.

I used to be a perfectionist. I'm not sure I owned it then, but people used to say to me: "You're so perfect," and the more I heard how "perfect" I was, the more upset I would get. I would react and say in a firm tone that I was not perfect! It also created this need, this feeling inside of me to live up to people's expectations. So, the more I was told how perfect

I was, the more I wanted to please, the more I wanted to do things right, the more mistakes I made and the guiltier I felt. I did not give myself permission to be human, to make mistakes. And I wore my guilt on my sleeve. I lacked healthy emotional regulations. People's opinions of me became more important than my own truth and my own well-being. I denied myself the right to be vulnerable. Being vulnerable was equal to being weak, and being weak was not part of who I am. All I knew how to do was to keep going.

What a vicious cycle I dug myself into. It made me feel upset and mad because I am not a perfectionist, it's just that I do want things to be right.

When I read Brené Brown's book, *The Gifts of Imperfection: Let Go of Who You Think You're Supposed to Be and Embrace Who You Are,* a book I'd read before and one we read at the Renewal Center, it gave me validation in a way. First of all, that I'm not the only one, that people like me do exist. We are highly driven, we are super achievers, and I know that something happened to us to make us this way. Brown herself admits that she has been a perfectionist in the past and that one of her challenges was to understand that and try to let go of it.

And it's not just trying to be your best, either. She says: "Healthy striving is self-focused: How can I improve? Perfectionism is other-focused: What will they think? Perfectionism is a hustle."

Brené Brown, who is a professor at the University of Houston and a PhD in social work, has spent decades studying the topics of vulnerability, perfectionism, shame, and other human emotions. She became very well-known after giving a TED talk in 2010 called "The Power of Vulnerability." Her social psychology embraces the idea that all emotions are valid and no matter how tough they are to own, numbing them has the effect of numbing positive emotions, too, such as love and joy. That we must be willing to be vulnerable, and that knowing ourselves, being aware, is the best way to connect to other people. And she comes from very personal experience, it's where her writing always starts.

You might recognize the trait that she and I share; all I knew was that I was very hard on myself if I ever made a mistake, and the harder I was on myself, the more anxious and depressed I got, and the more I was driven to be more perfect.

So, when I read her book, I realized that I could finally put a name to it, and start to be okay with it. Her research and this book spoke to me and gave me permission to be a perfectionist, in a way that is not as unhealthy as it used to be. Now, I do not strive for greatness in every part of my life – no, I admit that I'm messy in some areas, but if you open my kitchen drawers, you will see everything lined up, just so. That's one of many examples of my OCD. But I'm okay with that, PERFECTLY and I like that.

Why emotional health is so important

You might wonder why I chose emotional health as my second pillar, second only to sleep. It's because I know that whatever is happening with your emotions will somehow manifest in your body, whether it's as a migraine headache, back pain, ulcers, or even cancer. There is an undeniable connection between your emotions and your physical health.

And becoming aware of those emotions, being vulnerable to acknowledging them, and even talking about them in a safe environment, is one of the keys to health and happiness.

Often enough in our practice, families bring their children to the office with complaints of abdominal pain, headaches, and sometimes chest pain. After taking a detailed history and performing a thorough physical exam, we start to rule out a physical cause for their complaints and look at possible triggers for their symptoms.

And very often we find that trigger.

A patient of mine came in with abdominal pain and nausea. After taking a detailed history and physical exam, I discovered that recently the family lost a beloved maternal uncle to cancer. The young girl was close to her uncle but felt she couldn't grieve or show her sadness because her mother and grand-mother (who were present and crying during the visit) were sad. The girl didn't want to show them her sadness because she was feeling guilty about it. In her young mind, she needed to protect them. And by doing so the only way she knew how, her grief and her sadness manifested in her abdominal pain. I have many similar examples in my practice on how the children' emotional sufferings affect their physical health.

We pediatricians encounter this often in our practice, again, headaches and abdominal pain being the most common complaints. Lots of children who refuse to go to school in the morning because of a tummy ache are, in fact, victims of bullying. They might face other reasons at school, not doing well academically for one. They might feel inadequate, and that includes children with diagnoses of ADHD, anxiety, depression, and so forth. They just cannot keep up with the school curriculum, so they start to develop physical symptoms.

To me, this is a cry for help and we as professionals need to listen.

I don't like the term "mental health" because there's a stigma against mental health and mental illness in this country, in the world, really. And certain disorders are labeled diseases: We label anxiety as a disease; we label depression as a disease. How about we start to take care of our emotional needs, understand how we feel, and most importantly why we feel this way, then the journey of healing will begin. We will need to be mindful and willing to do the work. Start now right in this moment. Start where you are. I, by no mean denying mental illness however, I believe many emotional struggles are incorrectly labeled as mental illness.

And I also believe that stress is the root of manifesting many illnesses. It is huge, and it determines how well we are, whether we progress in life and manifest our desires and what's best for us, or we sink into dysfunction and illness.

How you show up in the world is a reflection of your upbringing. This is a very important, personal insight because I came from dysfunction. I grew up in a very loving but dysfunctional family. Of course, I didn't know it because they are so loving, and I definitely want to make that differentiation. There are dysfunctional families that are not loving, and there are loving, dysfunctional families. They just don't know that they are, and many people don't realize that they grew up in dysfunctional families. They just don't have the awareness of it, or they are in denial. The truth sometimes can be hard to absorb.

As children we observe and absorb, not until later in life do we become the observer and if we have the awareness and the tools, we can then choose what to absorb.

And that's why — while I am a pediatrician and my patients are children — my true target is families, my patients' parents, grandparents, and siblings. I want to give them the tools for change, what to unlearn, and how to unlearn what they grew up learning. My hope is they can acquire the tools and the awareness to navigate and create a loving, healthy environment for their kids to grow up in.

My family history

I grew up in a loving family, yet my parents had their own struggles and their own issues that they both brought into the marriage. Although both are wonderful and loving people, they had different personality types, which led to disconnection and miscommunication. This is what I observed and yes, absorbed, and this is what I brought with me to my own marriage and my other relationships.

It wasn't until my total breakdown and re-birth that I became mindful of this, but I was ready for it. In order for us to change, adapt and strive to become a better version of ourselves we need to be curious about it and ready for it. And I know I was. This is why I believe parents' awareness is so important for raising children who are emotionally and physically healthy.

Becoming aware

The first step is to pay attention to that feeling that something is off, follow your gut feeling, and follow that instinct. It's like when you meet someone, and something just doesn't seem right about them, something is off, and you feel uncomfortable around them. It's that innate feeling we all have. You can call it the source, you can call it faith, you can call it intuition. You just go deep within and ask yourself – *How does this make me feel? Does it make me feel good, or does it make me feel bad?* And then you follow that instinct.

Don't worry about making a mistake, we all make mistakes and go through things. If you have that awareness and follow your gut, you will become more attuned to what's happening inside of you.

Secondly, I am a big believer in self-help books, learning from somebody who has been through what you might be going through, someone who has done it and then written about it. I consider these authors my mentors and guides. We need to learn from people we connect with, either personally or through their work. They are our coaches through difficult times in our lives. We all can remember a specific teacher who had a big influence on us because they said something that resonated, we connected with them and can remember their words; they made us better people.

It's why we had required reading every night at the Professional Renewal Center. The best self-help authors have not only lived through what you might be experiencing, but they also have researched it and had other powerful influences. There are just goldmines of information that can support you in your quest for awareness.

HOW STRESS AFFECTS US

You know when you are stressed. Your heart pounds, and your body feels wound tighter and tighter. You get irritable, and everything seems impossible. The American Psychological Association (APA) defines stress as the "physiological or psychological response to internal or external stressors. Stress involves changes affecting nearly every system of the body, influencing how people feel and behave. For example, it may be manifested by palpitations, sweating, dry mouth, shortness of breath, fidgeting, accelerated speech, augmentation of negative emotions (if already being experienced), and longer duration of stress fatigue."[24] Chronic stress can cause or worsen conditions that include obesity, irritable bowel syndrome, heart disease, depression, diabetes, and asthma.

So naturally, you have felt stress. And you are not alone. The APA reports that, according to its 2020 survey, nearly half (49%) of American adults report feeling stressed. Most commonly, they report increased tension in their bodies (21%), "snapping" or getting angry very quickly (20%), unexpected mood swings (20%), or screaming or yelling at a loved one (17%). Granted, the APA stress survey was done in the midst of a global pandemic, and it estimates that "nearly 8 in 10 adults (78%) say the coronavirus pandemic is a significant source of stress in their life.

While older adults may have the life experience to know that things will probably get better, Gen Z (ages 18-23) are at a pivotal moment in their lives and feel they are looking at extreme uncertainty in their future.

You might know the term "fight or flight response;" acute, short-term stress is a defense mechanism. Our ancestors had to summon up a swift hormonal reaction to the threat of attack. The hormones adrenaline and cortisol flooded their bodies and mobilized energy to either fight the enemy or run like hell. The term stress was first described in the context of psychology around 1940 by Hungarian-born Canadian endocrinologist Hans Selye (1907–1982); so it is not just a modern condition.

Of course, in modern times you are more likely to confront an unreasonable boss, a cheating spouse, or an urgent email. But your body responds in the same way. And because the stressors we face today are ever present, we start to obsess about them, then we obsess about feeling stressed. What we need is a clean break.

---

[24] https://www.apa.org/news/press/releases/stress/2020/report-october

ACTION STEPS: STRESS REDUCTION

1. **Become aware** – Again, do a gut check: What is stressing you out right now? What's really going on? And what's the worst that can happen? In other words, don't run — stare the lion down.

2. **Calm your system down** – You might have certain go-tos that you know help calm you. I use yoga and meditation; you might need to stretch out in the sun and just breathe, read a book, or take a nap. Avoid drugs and alcohol, and instead try a three-minute meditation: Find a quiet comfortable place, close your eyes, and take a few deep breaths. Imagine you are breathing in calm and breathing out stress, and imagine a place you love being, maybe a sunrise or sunset. You will feel your body slow down and will be more able to release the stress.

3. **Look at your coffee consumption** – Later we'll get into details, but for now, limit the amount of caffeine you consume, it can really help you stay calm. Don't go cold turkey, which can cause its own issues. Just cut down.

4. **Get out!** – Studies show that vitamin D is essential for replenishing our adrenal glands, which regulate our hormone production. Get outdoors for 20 minutes a day (try for early morning or late afternoon), or supplement with 4,000 to 8,000 IU of vitamin D3 each day morning sun is more important.

5. **Try supplements** – Look for a good multivitamin that includes a B-vitamin complex, and make sure to eat foods rich in Bs like nuts, dried fruits, whole grains, and eggs.

6. **Exercise** – I rely on exercise to re-boot my brain; I bike, do yoga, and walk. Do whatever you like as long as it makes you sweat. It's a great release.

7. **Learn to say no** (boundaries) – Sounds so simple, but many of us have a hard time with it — and yes, women seem to be most affected, but anyone can feel the pressure to please people.

8. **Avoid energy vampires** and get rid of toxic people in your life; not an easy task to do but it makes you feel instantly better, with a weight lifted off your chest.

9. **Finally, put stress to work for you** — A little stress might help you meet a deadline or write a killer speech; just look it in the eye and make it yours. Be sure to set clear boundaries and feel the pride of a job well done. I did this while writing this book.

The power of self-help

There are people who have influenced and helped me greatly on my way to wellness. I've already talked about **Brené Brown** — she is a fantastic self-help author, one of the best. In addition to relating to her as a fellow perfectionist, I also love her message of vulnerability; in her book *Daring Greatly*, she writes about how having the courage to open yourself up can transform your life. Also, do check out her TED talk, "The Power of Vulnerability." It's easily found on YouTube.

Elizabeth Gilbert had a huge bestseller with *Eat Pray Love* — which I related to because she is a professional, was getting out of her marriage, and embarked on a spiritual journey. She inspired me to do what I love, and not feel guilty or selfish about it. And it's true — as guilty as you might feel about taking care of yourself and following your dreams, her book taught me that the people around you will feel it and appreciate it. They might not appreciate it while you are doing it, but they will. *Big Magic* is about how an idea catches you and you don't let it go; it comes back to you, and you must see it through. Gilbert believes that the universe gives you an idea and will provide a way for you to do it. This book, *Just What the Doctor Ordered,* is my dream, the idea the universe gave to me.

If there is one person I wish I had met before he passed, it's **Dr. Wayne Dyer.** He is my spiritual leader; he has had a tremendous effect on my life. And he has many books, but I think the most powerful is *Change Your Thoughts, Change Your Life.* How simple is that? How deep and accurate is that? He is all about teaching us that we are not our thoughts, you can choose your thoughts and your outlook on life and apply that choice to become what you want to be. You have the choice to think negative thoughts, or you can think positive thoughts. I try to follow that – when someone asks me how I am, I take a deep breath and answer, "I am great, I'm awesome, I'm having a great day," even if I'm not. I believe in energy, in good vibes, and that's what I learned from him over the years. I apply some of his principles in my practice. I used to tell my patients what I wanted them to do; now, I tell them that I am merely their guide, that I can give them recommendations, and suggestions, and they can decide what to do with them. I give them back their power. I especially love watching his You-Tube presentations, he was such an inspiring, calm, positive speaker.

This brings me to an important point: You might not be a reader of actual books. I don't always read books, many times I listen to them, or watch You-Tube videos of my mentors speaking. "Books on tape" are so accessible, podcasts you can listen to in the car, while you are working in the kitchen, or around the house. We are so lucky to have that access.

Nicole LaPera is known as "The Holistic Psychologist," and she specializes in childhood trauma; she's somewhat of an Instagram sensation. I like her because her teaching is very simple and very practical. She talks about what trauma is, how it affects our lives as adults, and how we can heal. She's kind of a new expert in the emotional health field, and another one I love to watch and listen to. She talks about codependency — I was a co-dependent person — and the importance of setting clear boundaries. You might not consider your childhood as traumatized, but Dr. LaPerla says: "Ideally, our parents are two self-actualized people who allow their children to be seen and heard as the unique individual[s] they are. The reality is that we live in a culture that does not teach conscious awareness, so most of us are born to unconscious parents ... repeating the same habits and patterns they've learned."

Louise Hay – the queen of spirituality. She passed in 2017 and I regret never having seen her, as well. She was so ahead of her time as a spiritual leader, and so powerful. Her presentations are timeless – her books are full of affirmations and simple techniques for healing from trauma, PTSD, and anxiety. Her voice is so soothing, many people use her meditations to calm their stress and even put them to sleep. She speaks a lot about self-esteem and learning how to love your body. She is priceless.

Here are a few of her affirmations:

- Whatever I need to know is revealed to me at exactly the right time.
- It's only a thought, and a thought can be changed.
- Everyone I encounter today has my best interests at heart.

Go to louisehay.com for much more.

Bestselling author **Lewis Howes** is a former Arena Football League (AFL) player whose football career was ended by a sports injury that actually opened up a world of opportunity for him. Now he has books, a YouTube channel with more than 2 million followers, and a podcast called *The School of Greatness*, and is one of my coaches. He is the best networker and entrepreneur I know, and his attitude toward life is absolutely inspiring. In his 2017 book, *The Mask of Masculinity*, Howes gives us permission to honor our vulnerability (especially men, of course) so we can create deeper connections and live a better life. I heard about his podcast from an acquaintance, I listened and immediately connected with his message. I had the privilege to be coached by Lewis and his team as part of the Greatness Coaching Program that was first implemented in 2021. I feel proud to be one of the founding members of the Greatness team. The main reason I joined the program was to learn the steps needed to write a book, as I believed by then I was at a good spot in my life. But what I gained was way more than what I signed up for. Lewis emphasized the need to concentrate on health, relationships, and then business. That changed my perspective and my priorities yet again. One of the most important lessons I learned from Lewis was how to hold myself accountable. This book came to life because of that program. I'd also like to note that I met incredible people during my time in the greatness coaching program, people who are deeply inspired to grow and to serve. Lewis Howes is the real deal, as good as it gets.

Dandapani is a Hindu priest who got a degree in engineering in his native Australia but left to become a monk under the guidance of Sivaya

Subramuniyaswami, one of the foremost spiritual leaders of our time. He writes and speaks about awareness and self-development. He delivers his messages in simple, inspirational speeches, and his book, *The Power of Unwavering Focus* is a practical step-by-step guide to understanding and harnessing the human mind. I listen to him when I meditate, or when I just want to be inspired by his words. He introduced me to the term "energy vampire," and how to deal with them. When you hear that term, you know exactly what it means, and we all have them in our lives — Energy vampires suck the energy out of you and leave you feeling exhausted. an energy vampire can be someone you just met for the first time or a close person to you who might be going through difficult time. typically this is temporary yet it can be draining while happening. But there are other people who I just don't want in my life. Here are some of Dandapani's quotes:

- The sleep factor is critical.

- What excuse do I have not to be <u>kind</u>? None at all.

- Be the person you needed when you were younger.

One of **Gabrielle Bernstein's** claims to fame is hosting the Guinness World Book of Records' largest guided mediation with Deepak Chopra. She is a modern spiritual leader in every sense of the word, using podcasts, Insta Live broadcasts, books, and appearances at conferences and on TV. She radiates beauty inside and out but is not afraid to let her own flaws and imperfections show as a way to connect with her community. Bernstein pulls much of her inspiration from *A Course in Miracles,* whose premise is that the greatest miracle is the act of simply gaining a full awareness of love's presence in one's life. I had the privilige of witnessing her powerful presence and words of wisdom when I attended the 2022 Summit of Greatness hosted by Lewis Howes in Columbus Ohio.

Thich Nhat Hanh I've already spoken about, and you'll read more about him as the book progresses, especially when we learn more about Conscious Breath. His book *Peace Is Every Step: The Path of Mindfulness in Everyday Life* is one of my favorites and one we were assigned to read at the Center. In it, he imparts such wisdom as: "Walk as if you are kissing the Earth with your feet." I love that. Also, "Fear keeps us focused on the past or worried about the future. If we can acknowledge our fear, we can realize that right now we are okay...." It's that simple. His soft, soothing voice is also a pleasure to listen to.

Everyone knows who **Oprah Winfrey** is, and there's a reason she has so much influence. She chooses wisely. For the book, *What Happened to You?* she partnered with psychiatrist and neuroscientist **Bruce Perry** to "explore how what happens to us in early childhood — good and bad — influences who we become. They challenge us to shift from focusing on *What's wrong with you?* or *Why are you behaving that way?* to asking *What happened to you?* In addition to the 2021 book, there are several videos available, including one made for the virtual 2021 South by Southwest. This one has a sign language interpreter on screen, which make it fantastically accessible.

I already have introduced **Viktor Frankl** and **Eckhart Tolle** to you in the introduction and I encourage you to read and/or listen to their work as you become more aware and start doing the work.

The work

The work is hard and challenging, it is demanding, and it is scary. And I consider myself a well-balanced individual (I am still doing the work!!)

Here's what I believe: The work is never done. It is not a project or homework. It is a lifetime commitment to be the best version of yourself and to always be happy in the present moment.

While I was writing this book, I had to take more than one break, I experienced some intense migraine attacks, physical pain, and intense sadness because some of the childhood memories that came to the surface made me realize I wasn't being honest with myself. I thought I was completely healed from my childhood trauma and from the toxic shame I carried with me for so many years. But I realized — when I couldn't write anymore — that I was still dealing with the anger, resentment, guilt, shame, and inability to forgive. I was still dealing with the trauma. All of those feelings I believed I had overcome, only to realize I didn't completely heal.

But here is what I knew for sure: I *was* able to identify my emotions. I was able to pinpoint the triggers and why I felt that way. Then I sought help from a professional. I now have the tools to recognize when I am not feeling well (physically and emotionally) and I know how to navigate through difficult times.

But it is most important if you want to really dig deep, become hyperaware, and really get into the trenches, that you find a safe environment in which to talk. One great result of COVID isolation is that psychotherapy became suddenly so much more accessible. Sites such as Talkspace.com, Betterhelp.com, and Online-therapy.com offer affordable, accessible sessions and tools to help you get started. Many insurance plans have behavioral health benefits, and colleges and universities often offer emotional health services for their community. You can also talk to a member of your clergy or a trusted friend; however, it is advisable to find an objective listener who is a professional and with whom you won't feel guilty about talking too much.

Please, if any of this work triggers you or you are hitting obstacles when looking for help, the SAMHSA (Substance Abuse and Mental Health Services Administration) offers a free national hotline, open 24/7, 365 days a year. 1-800-662-HELP, you can text 435748 (HELP4U) or TTY 1-800-4874889. And if you feel you are in the middle of an emotional crisis or you are a danger to yourself or anyone else, please call the National Suicide Hotline at 1-800-273-8255 or the new number: **988**.

THE SEVEN WARNING SIGNS OF DEPRESSION

It's not unusual for most of us to feel sad from time to time. Many have noticed the past couple of years — enduring pandemic lockdown, social and political turmoil, and possibly illness and death — have been particularly challenging. So, perhaps we all have felt sad, often.

But when feelings of loss, sadness, loneliness, a decline in self-esteem, and a general heaviness, become overwhelming and keep you from living your day-to-day life, you might be experiencing clinical depression. **Pay attention**

and be aware. What you are feeling is real and nothing to be ashamed of or embarrassed by.

The best place to start is with your primary physician, who can help identify your symptoms and help you manage them; they can also get you to a psychiatrist, if needed, and may prescribe medication.

Here are some signs to look for:

1. Fatigue
2. Insomnia, trouble falling or staying asleep, or wanting to sleep all the time
3. Trouble concentrating or making decisions
4. Crankiness or irritability
5. Pessimism and hopelessness
6. Lack of interest in activities that usually bring you joy
7. Persistent sad, anxious, or empty feelings
8. Overeating or loss of appetite

Some people experience the seasonal affective disorder, or SAD, a mood disorder in which people who usually are happily adjusted feel depressed as the days get shorter and darker. Many of the symptoms are similar to clinical depression, but often they can be reduced with light therapy — either simply going out into the sunshine or using a special lamp.

Prevention and treatment

Many of the therapies for clinical depression and SAD can also help prevent symptoms of depression, or ease mild blues.

Psychotherapy Talking with a professional trained to spot and deal with depression and depressive symptoms works well and often is prescribed in conjunction with medication.

Physical exercise has also been proven an effective prevention and treatment for SAD and most depression can be prevented or reduced with a regular, 30-minute daily routine of aerobic exercise such as walking or cycling, especially if you can manage to get outside.

Social connection Staying in contact with friends, family, and even acquaintances such as your local baker can keep the blues and even serious depression at bay. According to the American Psychological Association, nearly half of adults report feelings of loneliness, and studies have shown that a lack of social connection can be as hazardous to one's health as smoking 15 cigarettes a day, abusing alcohol or drugs, or being obese. Don't be afraid of appearing too vulnerable. Reach out.

Feeling a lack of family or friends you can reach out to? Try: joining a hiking group or choir; sign up for a crafting class; become a regular at your local coffee house; take up a group sport such as rowing or soccer; volunteer at a shelter or family clinic.

Medication There are many types of antidepressants your doctor might prescribe; many take a few weeks to work, and some have side effects, so patience with any therapy is key.

Crisis Counseling If your depression goes untreated, it can lead to extreme pain and possibly even suicide. If you or someone you know are experiencing thoughts of suicide, please call the National Suicide Prevention Lifeline at **800-273-8255 or 988.**

EMOTIONAL HEALTH ACTION PLAN

1. **Be aware** Notice when things are not feeling right with you; I know I keep saying this, but you KNOW when something is wrong. Pay attention and know that if you do not address emotional issues, they will surface in physical ways, and could manifest in conditions such as asthma, pain, migraine headaches, and diabetes. Know that when I finally found the curiosity and the courage to really examine my life

— going from feeling victimized to feeling empowered — my physical health improved too. It's all in your hands.

2. **Practice stress reduction** We all deal with stress. Go back to my stress reduction action steps and see if they help; if they do, keep practicing. At the very least, try the simple act of using one of your five senses: **See** what's in front of you, and really take it in. **Hear** the sounds outside, or in your space, tune in mindfully. **Feel** the breeze around your face, your body, and the chair you are sitting in, just pay attention. **Smell** the scents, fragrances, and aromas around you right now, even conjure up remembered ones. And **taste**, deliberately taste your coffee or tea, whatever you might be eating right now.

3. **Do a depression check** Do the warning signs of depression sound familiar to you? There might be just a few that do, and you might just be feeling a little blue. It's all valid. Use the action steps and see if any work for you.

4. **Be kind to yourself.** Science journalist Florence Williams did the research for her book *Heartbreak: A Personal and Scientific Journey* after her divorce caused her to lose sleep and weight, fogged her brain, and even brought on diabetes. Her research found that extreme heartbreak might cause actual physical changes, such as Type 1 diabetes, an autoimmune disease. It's fascinating reading and might help you be aware, accept and work on your emotional state much more gently.

5. **Stay socially connected** Social isolation is one of the consequences of our modern life, especially during a pandemic. Social media and Zoom calls help, but when and if it's safe, try to get some in-person interactions through dancing, crafting, volunteering, or finding a Meetup group that shares your interests.

6. **Get outside and exercise** Nature walks can work wonders for your emotional health, and exercise has a way of getting those feel-good endorphins circulating. Try for 30 minutes at least twice a week.

7. **Find help**. I also believe it helps to talk to someone, and if possible, a professional therapist, even if you are not sure what you're feeling. Online therapy is very accessible and affordable these days, and it might be better to talk to someone, not in your social circle with whom you can be completely candid.

8. **Heal the child within.** I personally believe this is the most important step, as we tend to carry our childhood aches and pains deep within. It is, however, extremely important to seek professional help, if possible.

MINDFUL EATING

"When practiced to its fullest, mindful eating turns a simple meal into a spiritual experience, giving us a deep appreciation of all that went into the meal's creation as well a deep understanding of the relationship between the food on our table, our own health, and our planet's health."

— Thich Nhat Hanh

"Let food be thy medicine, thy medicine shall be thy food."

— Hippocrates

> Refer to page 55 for your Mindful Eating quiz questions and answers.

I was a chubby child. I loved to eat. I ate when I was hungry, and I ate when I wasn't. Both of my parents were obese as well. They both struggled with their weight and talked about how they needed to lose weight and start to exercise, but instead, they just kept eating more.

My mother started to point out the way I looked, which started to affect how I felt about myself. I started to have issues with body image. I didn't like how I looked in the mirror. I cried when I tried on new clothes. I cried when the jeans didn't fit well, and I cried when I was called "fat".

So, I started dieting, My earliest memory of going on a diet to lose weight was when I was about 13 years old. It started as a bet. I did it by cutting down significantly on how much I ate and by walking. I wish it ended there. Even though I wasn't morbidly obese, the body image issues continued. It didn't help that society approved of "thin and tall," because I was neither. I am only 5' 2" and my weight hovered between 140 to 160 lbs.

The struggle continued, and that's when the purging started. Vomiting after especially heavy meals I thought was normal. I justified it by telling myself that my body will feel better if I get rid of the extra food. I truly didn't realize I was struggling with an eating disorder until many years later when I was told by a professional, "Dr. Katbi, most people go for a walk after Thanksgiving dinner. They don't intentionally throw up!"

Not until a few years ago did my relationship with food change. I still love food and I still love to eat. But I believe in moderation, not deprivation. I follow the rule of 80/20; 80% of the time I eat healthfully, and 20% of the time treat myself. I do not like to say that I cheated and ate junk food, I say I treated myself. "Cheating" has negative effects and makes us feel guilt. A treat is something we look forward to and makes us feel happy. To me now, food is medicine and just like the other pillars, it is so important to eat mindfully.

To eat or not to eat?

What you eat and how you eat can be extremely important to how you feel, how you heal, and how you feel about your body. Problem is, there is so much noise out there about the best way to eat, what kind of diet you follow, and even how you identify yourself.

Are you a vegan? Do you follow a keto plan? Do you eat gluten-free? Are you a flexitarian? Vegetarian? Pescatarian? The eating plan you follow can determine where you shop, who your friends are, and even who your partners are.

If there's one thing I think is most important, it is shopping for healthy, whole, fresh foods and making meals for yourself at home. Scores of studies have found that eating processed food incessantly can lead to many health disorders. Research also shows that fast food is not only unhealthy but also expensive, especially for a family. We'll take a look at what should be in your healthful shopping cart a bit later. But first:

How should you eat?

The United States food guidelines date back to the early 1900s when the USDA attempted to help parents choose food for their children, which evolved into a complicated "Guide to Good Eating" based on seven basic foods arranged in a wheel with no serving sizes. Then from the mid-fifties into the 1970s, the agency presented a "Food for Fitness: A Daily Food Guide," based on just four food groups — milk, vegetable, meat, and bread — but no guidance as to the consumption of sugar, fats, or calories. A revision in 1979 fixed that, and there were a couple of adaptations that led to the Food Guide Pyramid of 1992, by far the most comprehensive and visually interesting, and accessible, which included a variety of calorie levels and introduced the concept of moderation.

The problem with the Food Guide Pyramid was that its foundation was basically carbs, lots of carbs, which we now know are consumed in excess by most Americans. Users were left on their own as far as exercise, sleep, and all the other necessary factors for health.

Finally, in 2010 the USDA presented MyPlate.gov icon, with a goal of encouraging healthy eating, and a proportionate approach, not necessarily specific messaging or addressing again sugar, fats, or physical activity. Users can take a quiz and download an app to help them achieve their goals.[25] It can be customized or kept simple.

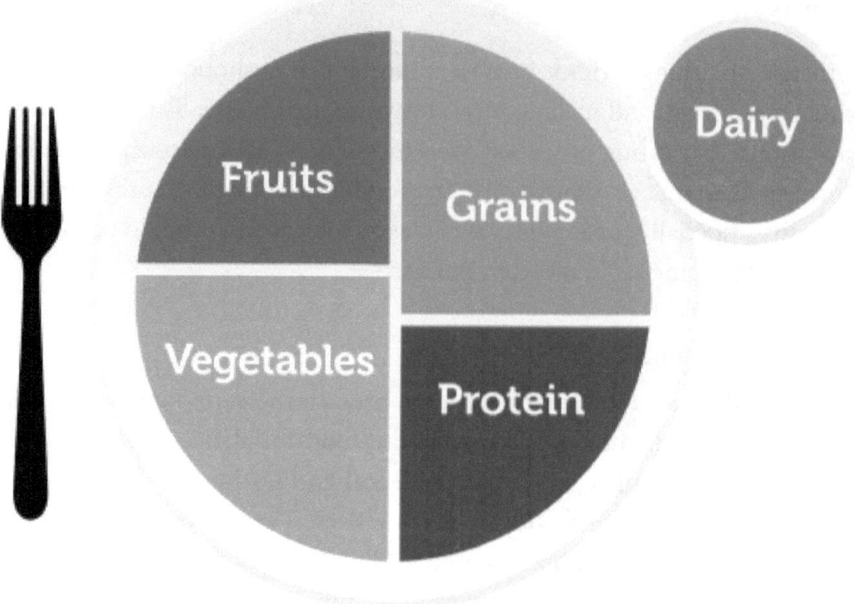

I do not promote any specific diet, but I definitely do *not* endorse the SAD diet — aka the American Standard Diet. In my opinion, it includes far too much sugar, too many processed foods, and high fat content, especially those hydrogenated fats that are just killers.

And I've tried many different diet plans, and found myself going back to this basic principle:

I like to keep it **simple and accessible.** We want to eat a healthy, well-balanced diet that includes the four macronutrients: Protein, quality carbohydrates, healthy fats, and fiber with lots of greens, different colors of vegetables, and fruit. For a few years — probably around three years —I didn't eat meat,

---

[25] https://myplate-prod.azureedge.net/sites/default/files/2020-12/ABriefHistoryOfUSDAFood Guides.pdf

I ate no dairy or gluten. I didn't have sensitivities, I just wanted to try it out. I ate fish. I never liked chicken much. That was not sustainable to me. But what we are finding is that moderation, yes, moderation, is the key. You can eat meat, or not eat meat, but it's not a good idea to eat meat three times a day, because of all the saturated fat and cholesterol that is not healthy. But once a week, once a month, have your burger or steak. Try to make sure it's good quality meat. If you indulge in bacon or sausage, look for nitrate-free, and again, keep your consumption moderate.

Limit processed foods: Read the label

Processed food can be packaged or frozen, and for the most part, it will have more than five ingredients and contain ingredients that sound like science experiments. Limit your consumption and eat them in moderation. But within reason: crackers, for instance, are considered a processed food, so try to find good quality crackers. And you might love frozen pizza; keep it moderate and watch out for added syrups, sugars, and hydrogenated fats.

Stay away from these big five ingredients if you can[26] [27]:

- **Sodium nitrate or nitrite** – is often used as a preservative in processed meats such as bacon, hot dogs, and sausages; studies have linked it to certain types of cancer.

- **High fructose corn syrup** – is a sweetener made from corn found in sodas, candy, juice, breakfast cereals, and snack foods. It has been linked to inflammation, diabetes, weight gain, and insulin resistance. Regular cane sugar, honey, or agave is much better as a sweetener, but I also believe that most Americans eat way too much sugar in every form. Limit your consumption and get used to drinking your coffee without sugar or artificial sweeteners.

---

[26] https://healthbeat.spectrumhealth.org/top-10-food-ingredients-to-avoid/

[27] https://www.eatthis.com/worst-food-additives/

- **Trans fat, or partially hydrogenated fats** – are fats that have undergone hydrogenation to improve texture and shelf life. Found mostly in processed foods such as margarine, baked goods, microwave popcorn, and biscuits, they have been shown to have negative effects on health including inflammation, which can lead to chronic conditions such as diabetes and heart disease. The easiest way to keep these fats out of your diet is to limit processed food consumption.

- **Artificial flavoring and coloring** – are just that: "artificial," and do not belong in your body. Some have been found to cause cancer or to be toxic to bone marrow in animal studies. Check labels and stay away from ingredients such as "chocolate favoring" or "strawberry flavoring," "red" or any other colors listed; look for natural ingredients instead.

- **Sodium benzoate** – is often found in carbonated drinks and acidic foods such as salad dressings and may be associated with increased hyperactivity. If combined with vitamin C, it may also form benzene, a compound associated with cancer development.

Quick tip: I read labels and personally look for the following:

1. Make sure there are no **saturated fats**, partially hydrogenated fat, or tropical oils.
2. No **added sugar**
3. How many grams of **protein** (the more the better)
4. How many grams of **fiber** (the more the better)
5. How many grams of **carbohydrates** (try to get no more than 20 in each meal)

Again, the easiest way to avoid these ingredients is to buy whole, fresh food and cook it at home. Now, to your ideal shopping cart:

JUST WHAT THE DOCTOR ORDERED: YOUR SHOPPING CART

I'm a big believer in **superfoods.** I have a few things I tell my patients and their parents that I want them to learn to love, to start eating them at a young age, and for the parents and caregivers to model for the children. Here's what needs to be in your shopping cart for optimal healthy eating:

AVOCADOS

Babies can start eating ripe, mashed avocados at four to six months, and continue as a staple in their diet through adulthood. Avocados are a wonderful source of unsaturated healthy fat and a good source of energy. They are a super accessible source of more than 20 vitamins, minerals, and phytonutrients, including potassium; folate; vitamins B3, B5, and B6; a huge source of vitamin C; and they also have lots of protein. They are easy to give to young children, you can put avocado in a smoothie, and you can make dips like guacamole with them. They are affordable and kids love them. [28]

BERRIES

Berries are super high in antioxidants, the compounds found in plants that inhibit oxidation, a chemical reaction that can damage cells. Berries are also high in fiber, which is necessary for blood sugar regulation and healthy digestion. Adults and children need at least 20 grams a day, but most only get about 15. A cup of raspberries gives you a whopping 8 grams of fiber; blueberries about 4, but what a delicious way to get your fiber.

---

[28] https://californiaavocado.com/nutrition/avocado-nutrition-facts/?gclid=CjoKCQiA3-yQB-hD3ARIsAHuHT64cAcg-AldQlMlQW-SGZTLQXxcimd1siog89uZR0TH19ZOorm3uMl-MaAvYjEALw_wcB&gclsrc=aw.ds

And they are packed with nutrients: a 35-gram serving of blackberries, for instance, provides 35% of the RDI of vitamin C, 32% of the RDI for manganese, and 25% of the RDI for vitamin K.[29] Experiment with putting into smoothies, oatmeal, and snack packs. Since berries are consumed whole and do not have a thick protective skin, try to spring for organic if you can.

VEGETABLES

Here's what I tell my patients and their parents about vegetables: Let's just say it — lots of kids don't like vegetables, so I tell them to try what worked for me. I used to make my kids a kind of salad bar and fruit bar, with cut-up apples, cooked carrots and spinach, pea pods, raspberries, and strawberries, and they got to choose what they liked. But they also had to try something new at least a few times, before they decided they did not like it. The other trick is to incorporate vegetables into smoothies or put zucchini into meatballs or pasta sauce, even pureed soups. What I also have found is that roasted vegetables, just tossed with a little olive oil and salt, are much tastier and kids will love them. Remember how we used to hate boiled Brussels sprouts? Crispy roasted Brussels sprouts are all the rage now. I grow basil and I make a pesto with all kinds of vegetables in it: mushrooms, cauliflower, carrots, and broccoli. It's always gone before everything else. Also, make sure there are plenty of different colors on the plate; think "like a rainbow."

LEAFY GREENS

Greens are essential for providing lots of minerals, vitamins, antioxidants, and fiber. And to tell the truth, the worst tasting ones are the best for you. Kale has come into big popularity in the last few years, but it is an acquired taste, and kids might not go for it; but try making kale chips: tear curly kale into potato-chip size pieces, toss with olive oil and salt, and bake in a 375-degree oven for 15 minutes or till they are crispy.

---

[29] https://www.healthline.com/nutrition/11-reasons-to-eat-berries#TOC_TITLE_HDR_5

I love arugula, arugula is one of my go-tos and this is the salad I eat every day at work. I actually crave it. If you can, here's where to spend a bit more and get organic produce; mostly because you are eating the whole vegetable, not peeling off a thick skin.

BEANS AND LEGUMES

Beans and legumes (peas, lentils, garbanzos, peanuts) are underestimated superfoods. I like all kinds of beans; I eat tons of hummus; we make lots of minestrone soup at home. Beans are full of protein, iron, and fiber and they also help with satiety because they have so much fiber in them, that you will feel full. You can add them to salads, too. You can soak dry beans before cooking, or using canned beans is fine, just make sure to rinse them to get rid of the excess sodium.

MEAT AND FISH

In general, buying organic and very fresh meat and fish from a butcher or grocery that you know and trust is best. I love fish. Families get confused about fish because of the messaging around tuna and mercury. But once or twice a week, have fish as your main source of protein. Just limit the servings of tuna and other large species. I don't love chicken, but I know it is a very popular and affordable meat. Just make sure it's well cleaned and fresh.

COFFEE AND TEA

Just like any food, coffee and tea can be good for you, or bad for you. Coffee and tea contain caffeine, which boosts mental alertness and may improve gut health and reduce the risk of Type 2 diabetes. In fact, some studies show a slightly reduced risk of premature death for regular coffee drinkers. Sometimes a cup of coffee can reduce a headache.

But caffeine can be your best friend or your worst enemy: Studies also show that drinking more than 4 cups of coffee a day can be harmful, causing anxiety, irregular heartbeat, and insomnia. [30] Best to not drink caffeinated drinks at all past 1 p.m.

And of course, if you get your coffee at Starbucks or Dunkin Donuts and fill it up with sugar and cream the calories can soar up to 680-1,000. But black, organic coffee can be quite healthful.

Here are my recommendations for caffeine consumption: Younger than 12 years old: no caffeine at all; 12 to 18 years old: 200 mg of caffeine daily; over the age of 18: 400 mg daily.

The average cup of Joe contains between 95 and 200 mg of caffeine (much more in some brands; for example, a 16 oz. grande cup of Starbucks drip coffee contains 330 mg).

A decaffeinated cup of coffee contains between 2 to 14 mg of caffeine, so you can still enjoy your favorite drink and have coffee dates with your friends without getting the rush and the undesired side effects of drinking too much caffeine.

And caffeine is not only present in coffee. Here's a list of foods and beverages containing caffeine:

- coffee and espresso
- tea; black, green, iced, or hot
- energy drink
- sodas
- coffee liqueur
- dark chocolate-coated coffee beans
- dark chocolate
- chocolate cake with frosting
- hot chocolate made from cocoa powder

---

[30] https://www.webmd.com/vitamins/ai/ingredientmono-980/coffee

EGGS AND DAIRY

In the past, conventional wisdom did not recommend eating eggs; now they are considered an almost perfect food.[31] In addition to having lots of Omega-3, protein, amino acids, and hard-to-get nutrients like choline, and the eye-healthy antioxidants lutein and zeaxanthin, eggs provide phospholipids for our brains. They are my favorite breakfast for children. Eggs are another place to go organic, preferably pasture raised if you can. And high-quality organic milk should be in your cart. Yogurt, yes, and I recommend full fat with no sugar added. There are so many brands promoted as healthy, but once you read the label you realize that many are not so healthy and need to be avoided especially in young children; they contain lots of sugar and unhealthy additives to make them taste better.

The American Academy of Pediatrics recommends whole milk in the second year of life, 12 to 24 months, due to the need for fat for rapid growth and brain development; after that, the recommendation is to use low-fat or fat-free milk.

As for yogurt, I still recommend whole-fat yogurt, or if you buy low-fat make sure you get the "no sugar added and no other additives." More often "low fat or fat-free" are loaded with additives such as salt, sugar, and chemical fillers that make them less than healthy.

HONEY AND MAPLE SYRUP

I recommend that people stay away from refined sugar, with an eye toward moderation. I drink hot chocolate during the holidays, for instance, but too much sugar has been linked to excess weight, heart disease, Type 2 diabetes, and even cancer. The biggest culprit in the U.S. is sugary drinks. While we need good carbs for energy, too much sugar can be very unhealthful.

---

[31] https://www.healthline.com/nutrition/10-proven-health-benefits-of-eggs#TOC_TITLE_HDR_11

And there are alternatives. Honey, for instance, and organic maple syrup or agave. Stay away from table syrup, which has lots of sugar in it. Stick with pure maple syrup. I love honey and I recommend using local honey because it helps with allergies, colds, and sore throats. Add it to yogurt or pancakes, or coffee and tea.

NUTS AND NUT BUTTERS

Nuts are an awesome food, and another you can make healthy or unhealthy. Moderation is key, and I recommend unsalted nuts for snacking; they are a good energy snack a source of good fat, and full of nutrients such as magnesium and protein. I throw them into my salads for crunch and variety, but I do stay away from the sugary, spicy ones, and also you must be aware of their salt and sugar content. I use sunflower seed butter instead of peanut butter.

And I caution my patients: You don't have to buy organic but do read the label and make sure you are getting peanut "butter" and not "spread." The spreads tend to have lots of sugar and hydrogenated oils, which are not good for us.

GOOD QUALITY OILS

Just the other day I discovered that Rachel Ray has trademarked the abbreviation "EVOO" [TM] for extra-virgin olive oil; that's how much awareness and popularity good quality olive oil has garnered. A good rule of thumb for buying olive oil is to always buy it in darker glass containers. The darker the glass, the better the oil. And while olive oil is good, so is avocado oil, and so is grapeseed oil for cooking. I use grapeseed oil when I make popcorn — I don't buy microwave popcorn because of the hydrogenated oils in it.

WHOLE GRAIN BREAD

Bread is definitely a good food that can be made bad. A peanut butter sandwich can be super healthy, or it can be garbage. Make it on white bread with peanut butter spread and tons of jam, and it's not so healthful. But switch to a seedy, nutty, whole-grain bread (make sure to look for those words, "whole grain," not just multi-grain), some fruit like banana or a no-sugar-added fruit jelly to sweeten it, and you have a much better version. I like to add grated carrot for sweetness. There even are awesome nut butters like almond and hazelnut that make the sandwich special. Do look for bread that is full of texture from seeds and grains.

HEALTHY SNACKS

Here is what I tell parents: Healthy snacks are fresh fruits, vegetable sticks (carrots, celery, bell peppers), unsalted nuts and full-fat yogurt with no sugar added.

To get this right, you do have to think ahead and buy carrots, celery, apples, kiwi, bananas, natural or organic peanut butter or other nut butters, cheese sticks, and unsalted nuts for older children, a small amount of dark chocolate for adults.

And I divide snacks into **healthy, fun,** and **junk** categories. Healthy is what I suggest above. Fun snacks are popcorn, pretzels, some snack bars (definitely only a very few), Chex mix (make your own, not store bought), and dried fruits.

Junk snacks are everything else.

Presentation is very important to children. Having a platter of cut-up fruits or veggie sticks with dips (peanut butter, hummus, guacamole) is a great way to attract hungry children after school and keep them out of the pantry. Pantry food is convenient and easy to grab, and it's usually where the processed snacks are. So, avoid having so many bagged or boxed snacks in the pantry.

And I personally love olives, another superfood. I buy packets of olives, put them on salads I make with Arugula and gorgonzola cheese, and I also eat them by the handfuls.

SALAD DRESSING

You really don't need to buy salad dressing. You can make the best dressing with your good quality olive oil and lemon. I like to add extras such as balsamic vinegar, mustard, and honey.

SUGARY DRINKS

When I ask children in my practice, "What are the healthy drinks for our bodies?" answers range from juice to chocolate milk to Gatorade, lemonade, iced tea, water, and milk. The answer I always hope for is water first and milk second. Milk does have natural sugars which makes it a sugary drink. At the same time, milk also has calcium, protein, and fat and it's fortified with Vitamin D, which plays an important role in growth, especially bone growth.

Let's face it: sugary drinks taste good, especially to young children. This is why avoiding introduction is the best strategy. The AAP recommends no juice or any other sugary drink in the first year of life and no more than 4 ounces of 100% fruit juice from 1 to 3 years of age, 4 to 6 ounces for children 4 to 6, and 8 ounces for children 7 through 14. However, we still encourage parents to avoid juices and other sugary drinks and instead focus on whole fruits and water.

I do get asked: "Is 100% fruit juice healthy?" I don't believe it is. It's always best to give whole fruits. And: "Is diluting juice better for young children?" Again, the answer is not necessarily. I personally do not recommend it and I believe dentists agree with me.

And you also don't need sugary sports drinks unless you are an athlete working out for 90 minutes or more in 90-degree weather. Or if you are a cheerleader, dancer, or football player, or you have low blood pressure or vasovagal issues. These drinks not only have about eight teaspoons of sugar per bottle, but they also are packed with phosphates, which strip the calcium from your teeth and bones, and may make you more likely to develop osteopenia or osteoporosis later in life. I don't drink them, and I don't serve them.

WATER

Let's talk about water. I do not believe in drinking tap water, but I also don't think you need to buy all your water at the store. Spring water is great if you can afford it, but I also love a good filtration system that filters out the toxic elements in many municipal water systems, but that retains fluoride. It's very important that kids and adults get fluoride. And try to use glass instead of plastic bottles; If you are using plastic, look especially for bottles that are BPA-free.

The topic of how much water you need gets a lot of play, but my rule of thumb is that you should drink half your body weight in ounces of water. So if you weigh 130 pounds, you should drink about 65 ounces of water a day. I also tell patients to look at their urine. Your pee should be clear and not too yellow. The recommendation of drinking eight (8) glasses of water daily has no background and I'm not sure how it started.

Remember that fruits and vegetables have a lot of water in them, so you might be getting plenty – that's when the urine color is key. Cucumbers, watermelon, and lettuce, all have tons of water in them; that's why I like the pee color test.

The benefits of drinking water:

- weight loss
- better physical performance
- helps treat headaches
- more regular bowel movement
- decreased risk of kidney stones
- better energy level
- helps prevent hangover

I drink water with a slice of lemon every morning, and I also like to keep a bottle of water that's infused with lemon, ginger or cucumber, or berries in the fridge, so it's easy to reach for instead of sodas.

JUST WHAT THE DOCTOR ORDERED: SUPPLEMENTS

You've heard this a thousand times: It's tough to get all the nutrients you need every day, and good supplements can fill the gaps in your diet. Here are some I recommend:

Vitamin D – I recommend Vitamin D to everyone because it doesn't matter if you live in Miami, as most people are not out in the sun all day. If you are, then you are wearing sunscreen to protect your skin. We know it's best to get sun exposure in the morning when it's not so strong, but even people in California and Florida are Vitamin D deficient. Vitamin D 3 is essential for bone health, oral health, heart health, and immunity. **How much:** For infants and children, I recommend 400 units per day, and it goes up as they get older. I personally take 5,000 units of Vitamin D3 in gel caps every day, and I'll double that if I feel I'm getting sick.

Omega 3/fish oil – I recommend using drops for fish oil. A high-quality fish oil is good for anyone, for brain function and heart health. **How much:** I started taking anywhere between 1,000 and 2,000 milligrams, and I notice a huge difference in my concentration and memory.

Probiotics – Probiotics promote healthy bacteria and yeast in your digestive system. The health of the microbiome in your gut is essential for your immune system and possibly even your mental and emotional health. **How much:** Follow label directions. A good probiotic should have several strains and more than one strain of bacteria about 20 billion units per dose.

Magnesium – I take magnesium before I go to bed, which is awesome because many of us also are magnesium deficient. It's great for muscle relaxation and sleep and helps with constipation. It can help ease headaches, too. **How much:** Try using anywhere between 100 and 300. A nice way to take it is a powder mixed with water.

Glucosamine and collagen peptides — Glucosamine is a chemical that helps maintain the health of the cartilage around your joints, so it's good if you experience arthritis or any joint pain, or are getting older. **How much:** The recommended dose is 500 milligrams per day. Collagen is used to keep your hair, skin, and joints healthy, and peptides are small particles that are easily digested. **How much:** Follow label instructions.

Peppermint capsules — I suffer from irritable bowel syndrome (IBS) and taking gel peppermint capsules helps. They also work better than antacids to relieve bloating and flatulence because they help relax the muscle wall of the bowel. **How much:** Best to take 1 or 2 capsules about an hour before meals.

ALCOHOL

Of course, the best thing for our health is to not drink alcohol. But we are a drinking society, and it's part of our culture to go out for a drink with friends. We know alcoholism is an issue that got worse during the COVID lockdowns, so again, look for the signs of a problem, and remember that moderation is key. And there are ways to drink smarter.

According to both the American Heart Association and the Academy of Nutrition and Dietetics, men should have no more than two drinks per day, and women should have no more than one drink per day. Excessive alcohol use is defined as drinking more than three drinks per day for men or women. A serving size is equal to 12 ounces of beer, 1.5 ounces of spirits, or 5 ounces of wine.[32] Studies have shown some benefits to drinking alcohol, especially red wine, but that doesn't mean you can go all out. It's best to drink clear alcohol with clear, sugar-free mixers, say vodka over ice with a lemon. And

[32] https://my.clevelandclinic.org/health/articles/16728-alcohol--your-heart-health

take breaks between drinking days — drink one day, for instance, then don't drink any alcohol for three days. That gives your liver time to detox.

We also know that when you drink, it's better to consume some fat such as cheese and crackers or nuts to slow down the metabolism of the alcohol, and don't drink on an empty stomach. Have some room temperature water with your drink.

FOOD ALLERGIES

I don't know about you, but the term "food allergy" strikes terror in the hearts of many parents. And so until very recently we used to tell parents to not introduce foods that may cause allergies, such as peanuts and eggs, until after a certain age in some practices, not until about three years old.

Everything has changed in the past few years; several observational studies have suggested that early introduction of potentially allergenic foods may be associated with a decreased risk of developing food allergies. Now we recommend slowly introducing foods that are known to cause allergies early in life to help *prevent* the development of allergies. The theory is the earlier you introduce, for instance, peanut butter or powder, between four and six months, the more likely the body will develop a tolerance to the allergens in it. Working with a health care professional is highly recommended if you are concerned about potentially allergenic foods.

NAVIGATING THE GROCERY STORE

You might have heard this hack before, but it really works:

Start at the periphery of the supermarket, then work your way into the center aisles. The reason is that the fresh foods — fruits and vegetables, salads, meats, and fish — are always on the outside aisles. So, fill your cart up with those necessities, then go to the inner aisles to get pasta, oatmeal, and cereals. As they were growing up, my kids hardly saw the juice or pop aisles. I just avoided them.

And I prefer going to smaller, local stores. I feel that the smaller the store, the better it is, and you might be supporting a family business. Also, if you shop at a big supermarket, you might be tempted to buy things you don't need. In a smaller store, you go in for what you need and you're out. Done.

Basically, I am recommending home-cooked meals instead of fast or frozen dinners. Frozen fruits and vegetables are fine, in fact, I recommend them to my patients, as long as they aren't full of too much added salt, sugar, or preservatives.

Spend as much as you can on quality food, organic if you can afford it, but any of the foods I recommend. Some families avoid berries and avocados because they are costly. I get it — I didn't eat a berry until I was 18. But it's better to spend money on high-quality foods because that's money you might not have to spend on doctor bills. And not everything has to be labeled "organic." Look for "natural", and "non-GMO", because they will be of higher quality.

I also really do recommend a food delivery such as Instacart or Hello Fresh, or even Imperfect (which sells overstock and not-so-pretty foods) because you can get good deals, and you are not roaming the aisles picking up stuff you don't need. You buy what you need for the meals you have planned, and there is not as much temptation as if you went to the store.

THE THREE-MEAL-A-DAY MYTH

There was a time, back in the 60s or 70s, when three full meals, breakfast, lunch, and dinner, were the norm, and if you stick to those three meals a day, you're not going to be overweight. But then snacking and shift work happened. Kids came home from school and went to the pantry and ate what they could find, usually processed, packaged food, chips, twists, and Cheetos. And then ate again when Mom came home to make dinner, possibly bringing home fast food for dinner.

For children, I definitely do not recommend intermittent fasting and yes, breakfast is the most important meal of the day. For adults maybe not so much anymore. Even though I stated earlier that I don't endorse any specific diet, there is evidence that intermittent fasting can be beneficial for adults over the age of 17. Try experimenting with eating later in the day, and possibly just lunch and supper, and see how it suits you. I also do not recommend eating late at night. You need at least two hours after eating before you go to bed, so try to have your last meal around 5 p.m. to 7 p.m.

PANTRY PICKY KIDS

Kids are very smart, they eat what their body needs. However, they learn at an early age that the pantry is the fastest and easiest place to get the carbs, fat, and starch they crave. We buy so many packaged foods such as crackers and cookies which makes it easy to go straight to the pantry unless you have a fruit and vegetable platter ready for them when they get home from school. Yes, I had the luxury of having a babysitter. But you and your partner can prepare a pretty platter with nuts and cheese and fruits and vegetables — remember it's all about presentation — and leave it in the fridge or on the kitchen counter so the kids have something they can grab to snack on when they come home, something that won't fill them up too much before dinner. Encourage them to not eat after a certain time, and to drink lots of water as they do their homework.

And don't forget to model that kind of healthy snacking for them as well. They will notice.

MINDFUL EATING ACTION PLAN:

1. **Make your own meals.** Use fresh, whole foods whenever possible. The simpler the better.

2. **Have a plan.** Bring a list and fill your cart with superfoods before anything else.

3. **Start at the periphery of the store.** Buy fruits, vegetables, and proteins before you dive into the interior aisle.

4. **Choose quality over quantity.** Know that if you spend a little more on quality, even organic food, you might need to spend less on medical bills.

5. **Plan healthy snacks for yourself and your kids.** Prepare fruit and vegetable platter to keep in the fridge.

6. **Invest in a water filter.** Learn what's in your local tap water and find a model that filters those toxins out.

7. **Use a food delivery service to save time and money.**

8. **Learn how to read food labels.**

INTENTIONAL BREATH

"When people ask me what the most important thing is in life, I answer: 'Just breathe.'"

—Yoko Ono

"To meditate with mindful breathing is to bring body and mind back to the present moment so that you do not miss your appointment with life."

— Thich Nacht Hanh

Refer to page 55 for your Intentional Breath quiz questions and answers.

*I*n a very short YouTube video Thich Nhat Hanh, the late Buddhist monk renowned for his teaching of simple breathing exercises, introduces one of them, saying in his gentle, soothing voice: "There is a text called 'Mindfulness of Breathing,' in which the Buddha proposed 16 exercises on mindful breathing." He goes on to say, "It's very practical. And everyone can do it. Not complicated. And you can already notice the effect of the practice after one or two hours..."

Basically, it's this: Notice your "in" breath and your "out" breath... "Breathing in, I know this is an in-breath," he instructs, "breathing out, I know this is an out-breath. So simple... be aware of in-breath and out-breath," and he writes this on a whiteboard. "As you breathe in, you become your in-breath only, the only object of your mind...." And so on. "If you are truly focused on your in-breath, you release everything. You release the past, you release the future, your projects, your fear, and your anger, because the mind has only one object at a time.

"Breathing in, I know I am breathing in ... and you become free." He goes on, "There is sorrow in the past, anger in the past; there is fear in the future..." and if you focus only on your in-breath for one or two seconds, you have freedom. "And if you have a decision to make, it's better to have enough freedom to make it; you are not under the influence of anger or fear." He smiles, and says, "And it is pleasant to breathe in." [33]

All I can say when I watch or listen to this amazing human being is, "Wow." And I want to share his wisdom with you.

The benefits of intentional breathing

I remember being a senior in high school, and it was during finals week. I thought I had done badly on an exam that could determine what university I could attend. In shock, I remember first holding my breath, then hyperventilating — taking shallow frequent breaths — leading to light-headedness and finally collapsing in my mom's arms. This reaction is actually common with teenagers, especially girls. A few of my own patients have been diagnosed with pseudo seizures (uncontrollable episodes of shaking) followed by syncope (passing out). Imagine if we taught our children how to breathe with intention, how beneficial that would be in their time of need.

Before we get into different breathing techniques, I want to share the benefits of intentional breath. Some might say, "I breathe, why do I need to think about

---

[33] https://www.youtube.com/watch?v=O_iDaIAPrGo

it?" The truth is yes, we do breathe automatically. But there has been so much research that shows taking even just a few minutes to breathe with awareness can promote some amazing health benefits. Intentional breathing can:

1. **Soothe anxiety.** — A 2016 study showed that students who practiced daily mindful breathing experienced less anxiety and more positive thoughts than those who didn't. [34]

2. **Reduce depression.** — Research published in the journal *Mindfulness* also has shown that stress-reducing exercises that include mindful breathing and body scan meditation reduced depression and PTSD levels among veterans. [35]

3. **Lower blood pressure** — A 2021 study showed that mindful breathing and relaxation techniques significantly reduce blood pressure levels in people with Type 2 diabetes [36]

4. **Reduce pain** — Studies show that mindful breathing can reduce pain, enhance circulation and digestion, and improve balance and self-awareness. [37] All important for your daily health.

First thing: Morning intentional breathing

When you wake up in the morning, just take a deep breath, just breathe. Be aware of your in-breath and your inhale should be longer than your exhale. Do it a couple of times, and it will give you energy and the gratitude that you have another day. That's what I start my day with. I am grateful I woke up. You take that deep breath, that inhale that lasts longer than the exhale, and that gives you energy.

It's the opposite at nighttime, at night you slow your breath and your exhale, your out-breath becomes longer, slower, and more relaxed. And you become more relaxed.

---

[34] https://journals.plos.org/plosone/article?id=10.1371/journal.pone.0164822

[35] https://link.springer.com/article/10.1007/s12671-015-0453-0

[36] https://www.sciencedirect.com/science/article/abs/pii/S1550830721000914

[37] https://hemaware.org/mind-body/breathing-easier-mindfulness-techniques-reduce-pain

Intentional breathing is simply being mindful of your breath, being aware. We take breathing for granted, but we want to make sure we are not holding our breath, and our goal is to be able to continue to breathe even when we are facing difficult emotions. That's what we strive to do.

And it's okay to use your fitness tracker as a reminder to breathe. Many smartwatches have reminders to breathe, just one minute or 30 seconds here and there to do some mindful breathing. You could call it meditation but it's much simpler than that. Wake up, sit up in bed, sit with yourself for a few minutes, and take some deep breaths

Anxiety hack: the exhale relaxes

Here's what I recommend to my patients: If you are feeling anxious, train yourself to use your breath for calm. Always remember it is about using your abdominal muscles when you inhale and not your chest muscles. The longer the exhale, the more relaxing the breath will be.

Start with simple one-to-one breathing: Inhale for a count of five, then exhale for five.

If you inhale through your nose, then exhale through your nose or mouth. We focus on slow breath, not deep breath. Just keep it slow. If you want to sigh as you exhale, that can be releasing as well. So that's the first step, inhale for five, exhale for five. Again, it would be beneficial to place one hand on your abdomen to feel how the abdominal wall rises up with the inhale and goes down with the exhale.

Second, try what's called four-square breathing or box breathing: Inhale for four counts, hold that breath for four counts, exhale for four counts, then hold that release for four counts. Repeat that four times, which will be about a minute. Foursquare or box breathing is an extremely powerful practice, and wonderful to ease anxiety.

The 4-7-8 breathing technique is an ancient yoga breathing technique. You inhale for four counts, hold for seven counts, then exhale for eight counts. 4,7,8 breathing is a favorite of mine.

For younger children, I recommend the following: Imagine one of your fingers is a candle. Place it in front of your mouth and pretend to blow it out. Kids love this exercise, and I practice with them and immediately feel the relaxing effects in my own body.

In my practice, I will also crumple up some of the paper on the table, hold it in my hand and have my patient blow it off my hand. They love that because I make it playful, they laugh when it falls on the floor and I have to pick it up. I tell them that it's part of my workout for the day. I might use a pinwheel, or a straw and a cup of water so they can blow bubbles. I even tell them to imagine blowing up a balloon, if they know how to do that. I might have them pretend to be a butterfly, cross their arms and see their "wings" rise and fall with their breath. The point is that of course, they must inhale in order to exhale, but the focus on the exhale is what soothes them.

And the point also is that there are many ways to instruct children and adults, so you have to find the trick that works. By finding simple and fun ways to help parents and children practice breathing together we can empower our families to calm down an anxious child.

I invite parents to practice these fun yet powerful exercises daily. This might be the first lesson of mindfulness we teach our children.

That's why people come to me, and that's what I want to teach. I feel very blessed that my practice and I are popular in my geographical area. Not everyone connects with me and the way I do things, but many do, and they come to me because they want to learn. That's what prompts me to write this book because I know people are looking for guidance. I know I am always looking for guidance.

I have learned so much from my patients, I've learned more from them than I can ever give them, really. For instance, the breathing technique about "blow out the candle" was taught to me by a mother who has an autistic child, and she used it during an office visit to help calm the child down. It was a powerful lesson.

INTENTIONAL BREATH ACTION PLAN

1. **Start simple** – Do not be intimidated, if that is something you're feeling when someone says the words "meditate," or "mindfulness." It's as simple as noticing that you are taking an in-breath when you inhale. Notice that, then notice when you take an out-breath when you exhale. That's all you need to begin.

2. **Explore different types of breathing** – If you take yoga, you might do a specific kind of breathing that syncopates with your movements. Yoga Nidra is a practice that involves breathing and progressive relaxation. Kundalini yoga teaches something called "breath of fire", which is a kind of panting that you can use to fire up energy, and alternate nostril breathing, which can be calming or energizing. Experiment with different kinds of breathing. Pranayama breathing is becoming popular for its ability to increase mental clarity and energy and release stress. Pranayama is a Sanskirt word to describe the exercises. [38]

3. **Remember that a long inhale and short exhale will energize; a short inhale and long exhale will calm and soothe you.**

4. **Practice intentional breathing daily, make it a priority, and set reminders if you need to.**

---

[38] https://www.artofliving.org/us-en/blog/pranayama-yoga-breathing-techniques

PHYSICAL ACTIVITY

**The Three Ss: Sweat, Strengthen, and Stretch
"Exercise not only changes your body, but it also changes
your mind, your attitude and your mood."**

—Author Unknown

"The reason I exercise is for the quality of life I enjoy."

— Kenneth H. Cooper. MD

> Refer to page 55 for your
> Physical Activity quiz
> questions and answers.

The magic of movement

Growing up, I wasn't athletic. I liked to read and I liked activities that didn't require much effort. I started working out as a teenager to lose weight so exercise was a chore and not a joyful time. I pushed myself at times without proper training. I even ran the Chicago marathon when I was 37, without joining any qualified training programs. Even though I finished the race and truly enjoyed my achievement, I was left with a knee injury and unable to work out for two full years. All of that changed with the shift of my mindset from I need or have to do it to I *want* to do it.

In the mid-1980s, scientists began studying the effects of exercise on health, disease, and aging. [39] [40] [41] The results were astounding, and it's now a well-established and accepted fact that regular physical activity improves one's health and quality of life. Moderate, consistent exercise can prevent diseases such as diabetes, high blood pressure, heart disease, cancer, osteoporosis, obesity, and cognitive decline, and can promote emotional and physical health and longevity.

Here are some of the proven benefits of a regular exercise routine:

Healthy heart – Heart disease is the number one cause of death in the United States. Regular exercise, especially aerobic exercise, helps to manage blood pressure and blood glucose levels while decreasing LDL (the bad) cholesterol.

Prevention of diabetes and obesity – Exercise can help you maintain appropriate body weight and can help regulate blood sugar levels to prevent Type 2 diabetes and pre-diabetes.

Osteoporosis and arthritis – Regular, weight-bearing exercise such as walking and running helps strengthen bones and, along with proper diet, may prevent the weakening of bones over time. It's also one of the best ways to prevent and manage arthritis by lubricating joints and reducing pain and stiffness.

Emotional health – The benefits of the three Ss go well beyond the physical. Research shows that physical activity can reduce feelings of stress and depression, improve your sleep, enhance your mood and feeling of well-being, and increase your energy levels. [42] It's even better if you can exercise in

---

[39] https://www.ncbi.nlm.nih.gov/pmc/articles/PMC4365421/

[40] Holloszy JO. Exercise, health, and aging: a need for more information. *Med Sci Sports Exerc.* 1983;15(1):1–5. [PubMed] [Google Scholar]

[41] Bortz WM., II Disuse and aging. *JAMA.* 1982;248(10):1203–1208. [PubMed] [Google Scholar]

[42] https://www.nia.nih.gov/health/infographics/emotional-benefits-exercise

a group, which will strengthen your social connections. Research also shows that social isolation can be as deadly as smoking 15 cigarettes a day. [43]

Longevity — Research shows that people who exercise live longer than those who don't. And a regular exercise routine that includes cardio, strength, and flexibility training has been shown to boost your **quality of life**.

The Three Ss

Kenneth H. Cooper, MD, often called "The Father of Aerobics," did extensive research that resulted in the recommended prescription for exercise of 30 minutes at least three days a week.

I like to take Dr. Cooper's recommendation a bit further and ask you to consider the exercise triad of **"Sweat, Strengthen,** and **Stretch."** I believe these three principles present you with a simple way to think about your optimal physical activity.

Sweat

You might think of this as the cardio leg of the exercise triad. Find an activity you love that raises your heart rate, makes you sweat, and that you can do for at least 30 minutes. Walking is one of the best ways to achieve this: it's free and accessible, you can do it outside — which fulfills the time in nature so important to us humans — you can do it with friends. Some people like a brisk walk, and that gives you excellent cardio training. You can even walk off weight if that is your goal; just make sure your heart rate goes up by around 70 beats per minute higher than your resting heart rate.

Cycling, running, rowing indoors or outdoors, and even swimming (yes, you do sweat while swimming) are all excellent ways to sweat. Stair climbing is a great way to sweat in the wintertime. You also can take a dance or Zumba class; some throwbacks to the 80s-style aerobics and Step classes even exist. Dance with the kids, race-walk around the island in the kitchen or jump rope. Try

---

[43] https://www.hrsa.gov/enews/past-issues/2019/january-17/loneliness-epidemic

skipping. Anything you can do non-stop. There are even forms of yoga that you can practice that get your heart rate up. Look for classes in power yoga.

Another metric to gauge your sweat activity is bringing your heart rate up steadily until you are a little winded, but still able to talk. If you can't speak or sing, take it down a notch. You also can use the "Rate of Perceived Exertion" (RPE) scale, aka The Borg Rating of Perceived Exertion Scale: [44] During your activity, rate your exertion based on increased respiration, perspiration, muscle fatigue, and heart rate, on a scale from 1 to 20; a rating of 6 being no exertion and 19 "extremely hard." Someone who wants to engage in moderate-intensity walking, for instance, would aim for a 12 to 14 "somewhat hard" RPE.

There is a misunderstanding that one should not do cardio if they are looking to build muscle; nothing could be further from the truth. I was having dinner with a cardiologist at my hospital who is very active, and I told him my son was very interested in strength training and told me that he thought he should not do cardio because it ruins one's muscles. I was able to tell him that my friend, the cardiologist, says that it's important to stay safe and balance the two, and that the combination is better for overall physical health.

Strengthen

Strength training can be weightlifting, body weight exercises such as abdominal curls, pushups, pullups, squats or even using resistance bands. As I often see in my practice, people misunderstand the role of strength training and think that kids should not do strength training. We recommend that children over the age of 7 start with resistance bands, Therabands, as a way to start building their strength. (You can find Therabands online, and also easy and fun workouts on YouTube such as this Kids Resistance Band Workout with Cailin: https://www.youtube.com/watch?v=z7b-EIsWzSE)

As children grow into teens and adults, I have found they often love going to the gym and using free weights and machines, but don't forget that you can

---

[44] https://www.cdc.gov/physicalactivity/basics/measuring/exertion.htm

use your body weight as resistance, by doing pushups, pullups, and ab exercises. Planks are one of the best exercises anyone can do, strengthening your arms, shoulders, back, abs, and core.

And don't forget your lower body: Squats, especially yoga squats, lunges, and walking lunges are the best things for your legs and your butt. Again, you can search YouTube for instructions, motivation, and how to add some hand weights, too.

While most people think of yoga as a way to stretch and maintain flexibility, the poses also involve strength, especially in the legs, to hold dynamic standing poses, and the abdominals for many balance and twisting poses.

It's especially important to continue strength training as we age. Without resistance exercises such as <u>weightlifting</u>, adults over the age of 50 lose 15% of their muscle strength each decade, and those over 70 lose 30%, according to recent research, so seniors who do regular strength training may be able to remain independent longer than those who do not.

BALANCING ACT

Speaking of aging, especially as a woman, for me balance is super important, and anyone over the age of 40 should be working on the core muscles and doing exercises that can strengthen them. Consistently working on these muscles might even improve your balance as you age. You can find yoga poses such as tree pose or an easy boat pose, or simply balance on one foot, then the other foot. Pilates exercises help strengthen your core, very important for maintaining balance. Research shows that falls are one of the most frequent and serious problems facing an aging population, and a relatively slight fall can be potentially life-changing. Prevention should focus on bone strengthening as well as muscle function. Many hospitals offer fall prevention exercise classes that teach physical activities as well as practical interventions.

Stretch

I love doing yoga, and that's my main exercise for flexibility. But there are many ways to stretch different body parts. I like to suggest that you stretch every day, and most importantly after a workout.

Start with your neck, your shoulders, and arms, and go through different body parts. Stretch your back and your sides. Stretch your hips with a yoga pose called "Happy Baby." It's important to stretch your legs, especially if you use them in your other triads of sweat and strength, and be sure to stretch your calves and ankles if you run or walk.

While stretching used to be recommended post-exercise, research is now recommending that we stretch before running to help warm up the muscles, stay flexible and prevent injuries. *Self* magazine has a slideshow of 20 stretches for better flexibility that I like a lot; it includes a standing hamstring stretch and a stretch for the hard-to-reach piriformis muscle that can cause tight hips. (self.com/gallery/essential-stretches-slideshow).

I do still believe that stretching after a workout just feels good and natural. Target the muscles you've just used and be sure to hold each stretch for a nice, slow count of 10 to 20. Do not bounce. Here's a link to some stretches that will help you relax as well as increase your flexibility: https://www.verywellfit.com/relaxing-total-body-stretches-1231150.

In conclusion

Getting more activity into your life doesn't have to be a chore, especially if you have children. Engage in pillow fights or chase the kids around the house for fun. Make activity a family affair — my son often helps me deliver treats to different parts of the hospital, and we use the stairs instead of taking the elevators. So, we are carrying trays and working our legs, but also our balance. I use the stairs every time I do my rounds in the hospital. Using the elevator has become quite foreign to me.

And think of your week as a whole: Going to the gym three times a week is awesome, but you also need to get outside and walk, take the stairs to your office, and ride your bike to the store. Just move, try to move as much as you can. Use a manual can opener, for instance, or a hand mixer. Yes, park farther away from the store entrance than you are used to. Think of cleaning the house as a workout. Go on hikes. Garden. Some things are weather dependent, of course, but try to get outside and walk as much as you can, even in winter. The more you do it, the more you will start to crave it.

There has been a recent movement to eliminate sitting so long at our desks. Most of my staff now use desks that can be raised so they can stand and work. And I notice they are always moving, moving their legs, walking around. It's so much better for them.

PHYSICAL ACTIVITY ACTION PLAN

1. **Find a workout you enjoy** – You are more likely to stick to exercise that is fun for you. Do you like to run, but need company? Join a running group. Do you like to be on the water, synching into the rhythm of rowing? Find a rowing club. Did you love riding your bike as a kid? There are clubs for all levels of cyclists, too.

2. **Put your workout on your calendar** – Make exercise a recurring event and try different times of the day. If you get your physical activity out of the way in the early morning, you are done for the day. Some people like to end their day with a workout but might find it's easier to skip as the day gets busier. If you can plan to work out with a buddy, you are more likely to make that appointment.

3. **Set goals** – Rather than just vowing to exercise more, be specific: Make your goal to exercise for 30 minutes every Monday, Wednesday, and Saturday, for instance. Or set a goal of walking three miles every week. When you reach one goal, re-evaluate and set new goals to stay motivated.

4. **Check out your local YMCA** – The Y has classes for everything: Old-school aerobics, Pilates, yoga, dance, strength training, and calisthenics, too. Many have swimming classes and sessions for swimmers of all levels, even people who just want to walk in the water. Check out the nutrition, stress-reduction, and financial planning workshops as well.

5. **Plan ahead** – Put prompts around your house, or your car, such as keeping your gym bag within sight, at the foot of your bed, or on your passenger seat. Some people even sleep in their running clothes so they can jump out of bed and get out without a lot of fuss. Whatever works for you.

THE CHOICE IS YOURS

"Remember, you have been criticizing yourself for years and it hasn't worked. Try approving of yourself and see what happens."

— Louise L. Hay, *You Can Heal Your Life*

"You have the power to heal your life, and you need to know that. We think so often that we are helpless, but we're not. We always have the power of our minds. Claim and consciously use your power."

—Louise L. Hay

I want people to know that they can handle their own health, that they can make choices.

You are not your thoughts. It's the choices you make out of those thoughts that you have control over. And that's what I want people to know, that they are not stuck, they can change what they believe, they can change their beliefs, they can get unstuck. They can take care of their own emotional, mental, physical, and spiritual health. And they don't have to do it alone. That's very important. If I want them to be curious about it, I want them to, you know, learn how to be aware and make the changes they want to make, step by step. It's not all or nothing. It's a process.

I also want my work and my experiences to empower women.

It's interesting. I'm choosing to tell my story because I think some people will be able to relate to me, that I'm not just a physician, and certainly not someone people should be intimidated by. I'm a human, and I'm telling you my own personal experience and what I've learned from my work. I feel it's powerful because it's a combination of the two.

There are a couple more authors whose books have had a great influence on me. One is Lori Gottlieb, who wrote the book, *Maybe You Should Talk to Someone*, an instant *New York Times* bestseller about what she has learned as a psychotherapist who went into therapy herself when the man she was all set to marry unexpectedly broke up with her, "shattering her sense of the present and the future." She also writes a column for *The Atlantic* and has a podcast.

"Part of getting to know yourself is to **unknow** yourself," Gottlieb writes, "to let go of the limiting stories you've told yourself about who you are so that you can live your life and not the stories you've been telling yourself about your life." I find that so inspiring. Now, she has put out a workbook that uses those lessons as a guide for discovering and understanding our own stories. It's definitely a tool you can use to get unstuck.

James Clear, the author of *Atomic Habits,* is a journalist and writer who was severely injured when a high school teammate accidentally hit him in the face with a baseball bat. Despite the injury, he went on to be selected as the top athlete at Denison University and was accepted to the ESPN Academic All-America Team. After his injury, Clear began working on himself and became convinced that the quality of one's habits dictates the quality of one's life. He started with small, reachable goals (sound familiar?) and eventually became the person he wanted to be. He believes everyone has the same potential, and that it's not enough to break bad habits if you want to become healthier and happier. You have to find new, better habits.[45] "The most practical way to change who you are," he believes, "is to change what you do."

Getting Better

Something I want to leave you with is this:

It takes time. So, take your time. Be curious about your health and about your life, start to read and start to ask questions, start to experiment with a few things, and see what works for you. Start small and build on that. As I've said, I was incredibly lucky, blessed, really, to have been pushed into the Professional Renewal Center. And, I was pushed, but as it turned out, it was exactly what I needed, that complete immersion, that daily routine of writing, thinking, reading, and talking that finally took hold of me.

One of the things I remember, toward the end of my time at PRC, there was one day that was really nice and sunny, and I walked the main street of Lawrence, Kansas. I went to an ice cream shop and I bought ice cream, enjoyed looking at the people. I was actually smiling. I felt at ease, and I felt at peace. And I sent pictures to my children.

And I thought: *I'm actually enjoying my time here.* I realized that this is not a prison, this is just treatment, this is a life-changing event for me. And I was very lucky to have experienced it. I felt gratitude and I want you to know that you can get the same thing, if you want it and want to do the work. You don't have to enroll in a program, you don't even have to hit rock bottom. All you need is to use what you've learned here.

And it takes time. Even after I came back, I could feel that I was getting better. Then, some days I felt less better. I was not feeling as resentful as I used to, and or the victim, but I had to keep doing the work. And I started to see myself as being responsible for things that happened, and that I had a huge part in it. So, I admitted that, and took responsibility for my wrongdoing. I definitely was not perfect. And I took full responsibility for it. And those

---

[45] https://www.oberlo.com/blog/atomic-habits-by-james-clear-summary

changes afterward, took a while to be implemented, obviously. It's daily work and it's still working. It's a work in progress. I'm a work in progress. So are you.

Curiosity about alternatives

Even though I was trained as a medical doctor, an M.D., I believe in keeping any and all alternatives for healing open. I truly believe in a holistic approach to medicine, which means looking at and treating the whole person, taking into account mental emotional, and social factors rather than just the symptoms of a disease.

Alternative therapies and medicine that integrate with traditional, Western medicine have become much more widely accepted recently, and I'm a big fan. Here are some therapies I know can help with a variety of ailments:

Chiropractic medicine – About 35 million Americans see a chiropractor each year, and I am one of them. I have found that the work a chiropractor – a doctor who has earned a degree through four to five years of full-time study — does/can help with back pain, neck pain, and many Musculoskeletal problems in the shoulders and other parts of the body. **Best for:** Spine, neck, back, muscle and joint pain, sciatica. **How to find a practitioner:** Start with recommendations from friends and family or even your medical doctor. Make sure your medical doctor knows you are seeing a chiropractor, and that the chiropractor has a degree from a college accredited by the Council on Chiropractic Education.

Massage therapy – Massage therapy has been proven to soothe sore muscles, improve sleep, and ease stress and chronic pain. It has been used to help babies born prematurely gain weight and to ease the side effects of cancer treatments. Recent studies also show benefits for patients with fibromyalgia, depression, anxiety, and fatigue. There are many types of massage ranging from gentle and relaxing Swedish massage to energizing and results-oriented deep tissue and sports massage. **Best for:** Muscle, joint, and back pain, tension, stress, and insomnia. **How to find a practitioner:** There are no national certifications, only local and state certifications, and educational requirements vary widely. Get a recommendation, look for credentials such as L.M.T., N.C.M.T., C.M.T., and find out where the massage therapist went to school. Be sure to let your medical doctor know you are seeing a massage therapist.

Traditional Chinese Medicine Also known as acupuncture and TCM, this ancient technique is now practiced by medical doctors in the West as well. The practice involves, yes, needles that are inserted at key points along energy channels — called meridians — to ease many kinds of pain and balance energy. But acupuncturists also are educated in herbal medicine, which can be used as an alternative or complementary treatment. **Best for:** Acupuncture has been studied widely and has been found efficacious for many kinds of pain, including chronic headache, neck and back pain, and arthritis. It also has been found to be effective for depression and anxiety, digestive and skin disorders, chronic obstructive pulmonary disease, Parkinson's, and weight loss, and to ease side effects of cancer treatments. **How to find a practitioner:** Check credentials and education. Most states require an L.Ac. (licensed acupuncturist) certification. Call ahead for a 10-minute interview, if possible. Inquire up front about costs and if your insurance covers acupuncture (many do). Again, be sure to tell your medical doctor about your plans to seek acupuncture.

I'll repeat: When you are exploring complementary and integrative therapies, be sure to let your primary care doctor know, especially if you might be taking supplements or herbal remedies that might interact with your regular medications. Check out the requirements for certification and licensing in your area. Try to meet with the practitioner by phone or in person, to get a sense of their vibe, and how you might get along. Trust your gut: If anything doesn't seem right, go with your instinct.

A word about COVID

I cannot conclude this book without talking about the pandemic that, as I write, we are still struggling with. I have spoken to you a lot about stress and anxiety. The COVID pandemic and lockdowns have been all about those emotions, on many levels. It's being alone, it's being afraid, it's being uncertain, and then having to carry the load of work or school.

And, at this point (September 2022) we have emerged somewhat from isolation and I believe that's due to enough people getting vaccinated and getting boosters. But I, being a physician, have heard from people on all sides of that issue, from all walks of life, and I feel it's my duty to listen and to keep my mind open. I need to listen to patients who are not vaccinated and why they made that decision for themselves and their families. I want to know. I am curious, and they know I will not judge them.

But I also have the responsibility to call attention to things parents might not be seeing: the speech delay and other developmental issues, the additional screen time; when I enter an exam room, the parent is on their phone, the child is on their phone — and that has definitely gotten worse during COVID.

Mental health issues related to the COVID-19 pandemic are also more prevalent. The isolation, loss of income, fear, and bereavement are triggering mental health conditions or exacerbating existing ones, such as anxiety, depression, and alcohol use. A survey found excessive alcohol consumption was up 21% during the pandemic, which later can lead to a significant increase in mortality, liver failure, and liver cancer.

As I discussed in Chapter 2, burnout amongst health care workers is at an all-time high. It is real and it is frightening. I see it on a personal level in my own office and when I talk to other health care workers.

So, I listen to their concerns, my colleagues, and my patients, and call attention to the science, that getting vaccinated is the only way out of this pandemic and we need to do it to protect our children. It's not just about you and your beliefs. And my decisions are not just about me, they are about the community.

And I had COVID. Right around Christmas 2021, there was another surge in cases. I had a minor illness. I was fully vaccinated and boosted. And even though the illness was mild, the effect on me emotionally was not. We had to cancel our large family Christmas gathering, just as we had canceled Thanksgiving 2020, due to the anxiety of getting the disease, which was the common theme for many people.

Now more than ever, we need to be actively participating in our own health and wellness. We need to actively learn about what is healthy and good for us. That includes sleeping well, eating healthfully, staying active, using our breathing as a great tool, and most importantly taking care of our emotional wellbeing. One of the greatest gifts I learned is how to stay away from toxic people and how stress truly affects our lives. We do all that with the help of our family, friends, health coaches, trainers, and health care professionals.

My hope, my silver lining is that COVID will draw attention to the fact that people who are healthier and stronger are more likely to survive and thrive, either not getting the virus, or living through it and staying healthy on the other side.

Happy Ending?

I have not looked at the full report of my neuropsychological evaluation in many years, not until I started writing this book. Reading the report now when I am at a healthy point in my life, is very different from when I first read it.

Back then, I remember feeling angry, and strongly disagreeing with the team who did the evaluation and the diagnosis. I thought they were a bunch of idiots who didn't know what they were doing. I thought things like *who are they to know what I went through?* And *they don't understand me or my illness.* Things like that.

I definitely read it with the victim mentality. Of course, at that time I was going through so much pain on many levels —physically and emotionally — I was not able to navigate through the report mindfully. Reading the report years later is empowering in a way because I am in such a good place in my life, I know how much progress I have made, I am much more aware of my life and myself. I also know that I'm so much more than my illness, my illness doesn't define me.

I repeat: My illness doesn't define me. It is part of me but it is not who I am. I am not depressed, anxious, a migraineur, or whatever other diagnoses I had or have. A better way is to say, "I suffered from anxiety, depression, migraine headaches, and fibromyalgia pain."

It was during one of my earlier therapy sessions when I was feeling sorry for myself that a no-nonsense therapist told me: "Dr. Katbi, are you going to tell your patients who have asthma or diabetes that they cannot have a good life because of their illness?" She was one of the first therapists who helped me realize that I am indeed so much more than my illness.

I am not underestimating what I went through, the pain and sufferings were real and at times debilitating, I am simply grateful for where I am today and for being able to find my way to wellness.

Here, let me share what I was diagnosed with at the end of the full evaluation:

- **dysthymia (anxiety and depression)**
- **unspecified personality disorder**
- **mild alcohol use**
- **mild eating disorder**
- **chronic intractable migraine headaches (verified by a neurologist)**
- **irritable bowel syndrome by self-report.**

And my treatment goals:

1. Work through past relationships' difficulties and traumas
2. Be able to work efficiently without falling victim to somatic symptoms
3. Find a healthy connection with people instead of being overly concerned about "undoing" and "people pleasing"
4. Process relationship between chronic pain and stress

I do agree with all of those (mental health issues) reported in the final evaluation. Even though I saw many therapists over the years prior to the intense treatment I received at PRC, it was not enough. Not until I started to have a deep and true awareness of those issues, not until I worked on healing the child within.

Working on the family of origin and how that affects who and what we become, reading so many self-help books, applying their principles, and working with a group of professionals who were versed in such issues and traumas — that's when the true healing began. That is when I started to see results. Furthermore, not until I changed my own mindset from being the victim to being in part responsible for what happened in my life.

I moved from w*hy is this happening to me?* To – *Hmmm. I see those things are happening for me.* I know now that those were lessons and trials. I failed some when I repeated the same mistakes, but my gains are much more than my failures and that is why I'm here today declaring that I am well. I am healthy, I am loving, and I am grateful for all those lessons from the very tough and challenging ones to the life successes that came easy.

At the time of writing this book, I am still practicing pediatric medicine. I love what I do, I love helping families. I love watching the kids grow and thrive and I like being the guide.

I used to tell families what to do, now I tell them I am their guide and I make recommendations. I want them to be curious about it, learn it for themselves and take from it what works for their family. I guide parents and help them tap into their inner wisdom and empower them to raise emotionally intelligent and physically healthy children. No family is alike, and no child is alike; every child in my practice is unique and I approach every situation with that in mind.

I still work for the same hospital, I have great relationships with management and staff, and I voice my opinion and respect other people's opinions. I listen to my staff, and I respect them deeply.

A big lesson I learned from my own personal story and the burnout I endured is to be mindful of other people's burnout. Because of COVID, health care suffered greatly and healthcare workers on all levels suffered greatly, and my office was no exception. I earned my staff's respect by staying true to myself, addressing and acknowledging their pain and suffering through the pandemic and I listened to them with an open heart and open mind.

On a personal level, I am back to being the happy child I once was. My inner child is healed for the most part. At times some things, some of my issues, emerge but I can feel them, and I immediately look for triggers, I identify them and use the tools I acquired to navigate through them. I still seek advice from professionals when I feel the need to.

I truly believe in the five pillars of optimal health, and I hope you give them a chance. My goal is to help people explore these pillars; hopefully, they will resonate with them as much as they resonated with me.

I want to share with you my biggest win with all the work I have done so far; I consider this the biggest compliment a mother can receive. One of my children was asked who she admires and looks up to in her life. She paused and she answered, "My mom. She's learned to apologize for things she's said and done in her life and is constantly in pursuit of growth. She's always working to better herself. And I think that is really rare in a parent, or anyone her age. People want to stop growing at a certain point, and my mom has shown me it is never too late to say "Sorry, [to] grow, and have ambitions. She inspires me to always better myself."

Another one of my daughters recently called me a "trailblazer." She meant she saw me as leading the way, someone who is going places others might not. That made me feel proud, and to feel that I am inspiring my own children ... priceless.

That is one of the big reasons I wrote this book. You cannot turn the clock back, but you can always start again with healthier habits and healthier choices. It is, in fact, up to us to change our thoughts and our lives.

"Stop acting as if life is a rehearsal. Live this day as if it were your last. The past is over and gone. The future is not guaranteed."

— Wayne Dyer

"The two most powerful warriors are patience and time.

—Leo Tolstoy, *War and Peace.*

APPENDIX

Suggested Books

Bourne, PhD. Edmund. *The Anxiety and Phobia Workbook*

Bradshaw, John. *Healing the Shame that Binds Us*

Brown, Brené. *The Gift of Imperfection*

Chodron, Pema. *Start Where You Are*

Clear, James. *Atomic Habits*

Coelho, Paulo. *The Alchemist*

Doidge, Norman. *The Brain That Changes Itself*

Dyer, Dr. Wayne. *Change Your Thoughts, Change Your Life*

Gilbert, Elizabeth. *Eat Pray Love*

Gilbert, Elizabeth. Big Magic

Hanh, Thich Nhat. *Peace is Every Breath*

Howes, Lewis. *The School Of Greatness*

Frankl, Viktor. *Man's Search for Meaning*

Neff, Kristen. *Self-Compassion*

Nestor, James. *Breath*

Oldham, Dr. John. *The Personality Self Portrait*

Poijula, William. *The PTSD Workbook*

Ruiz, Don Miguel. *The Four Agreements*

Sapolsky, Robert. *Why Zebras Don't Get Ulcers*

Singer, Michael. *The Untethered Soul*

Smith, Manuel. *When I Say No, I Feel Guilty*

Stevenson, Shawn. *Sleep Smarter*

The Rumi Collection: An Anthology of Translations of Rumi
Richardson, Ronald Dr. *Family Ties That Bind*
Rogers, McKay. *The Anger Control Workbook*
Walker, Matthew. *Why We Sleep*
Davis, Martha; Paleg, Kim; Fanning, Patrick. *Messages.*
Paterson, PhD, Randy. *The Assertiveness Workbook*
Whitfield, Charles. *Healing the Child Within*
Winfrey, Oprah; Perry, MD, PhD. Bruce. *What Happened To You?*

Suggested podcasts

School of Greatness, Lewis Howes
The Model Health Show, Shawn Stevenson
On Purpose, Jay Shetty

On Instagram

Nicole LePera, The Holistic Psychologist
Lewis Howes, school of greatness
Power of positivity

On YouTube

Gabby Bernstein
Dr. Joe Dispenza
Dr. Wayne Dyer
Louise Hay
Eckhart Tolle
Lewis Howes

Meditation/breathing apps

10% Happier
Insight Timer
Calm
Breathwrk
Headspace